Volume Two

RADIOGRAPHIC ANATOMY and POSITIONING WORKBOOK

Steven G. Hayes Sr., BSRT, MEd, RT(R)
Formerly Assistant Professor
Department of Radiologic Technology
Midwestern State University
Wichita Falls, TX

with 184 illustrations

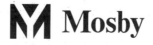 Mosby

St. Louis Baltimore Boston Carlsbad Chicago Naples New York
Philadelphia Portland London Madrid Mexico City Singapore Sydney

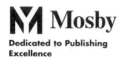

Mosby
Dedicated to Publishing Excellence

Editor: Jeanne Rowland
Developmental Editor: Lisa Potts
Editorial Assistant: Nicole Alexander
Project Manager: Gayle Morris
Design and Layout: Chad Reidhead
Copyeditor: Susan Warrington
Manufacturing Supervisor: Betty Richmond

FIRST EDITION

Printed in the United States of America
Composition by Wordbench

Mosby-Year Book, Inc.
11830 Westline Industrial Drive
St. Louis, Missouri 63146

International Standard Book Number: 0-8016-7980-X

96 97 98 99 00 / 9 8 7 6 5 4 3 2 1

DEDICATION

This workbook is dedicated to the most important person in my life, my wife, Sharon Hayes. Her love and support for me have created all the happiness in my life. She was the motivation that inspired me to become a radiologic technology educator, and she is the reason I still pursue goals; therefore, this publication is for her.

PREFACE

This workbook consists of various exercise items that review osteology, anatomy, physiology, arthrology, and radiographic examinations. This workbook has been developed to accompany *Mosby's Radiographic Instructional Series: Anatomy, Positioning, and Procedures* and *Merrill's Atlas of Radiographic Positions and Radiologic Procedures*. The major chapters of this workbook are divided into two sections: (1) An anatomy section and, (2) a positioning section. The anatomy sections consist of various exercises that may include diagrams, direct questions, matching exercises, and crossword puzzles. The positioning sections include questions, statements, and radiographs that refer to standard radiographic projections. The last exercise is a collection of multiple-choice questions to review the entire chapter. All answers for exercises are found at the end of each volume.

Some of the radiographic projections described in *Merrill's Atlas* are included for reference purposes only and are no longer routinely performed in radiologic imaging facilities. Therefore, we have chosen to focus on essential terminology, anatomy, and positioning information for the projections identified as necessary for entry-level competency as determined by a survey of radiologic technology programs in the United States and Canada. For more information on the survey, consult the Preface contained in *Merrill's Atlas*.

Some chapters of *Merrill's Atlas* (Volumes 1 and 2) have limited radiographic applications, or are comprised of radiographic procedures only rarely performed today because of technological advances in adjunct medical imagery modalities (e.g., computed tomography; magnetic resonance imaging; diagnostic ultrasound). Because those chapters do not include radiographic examinations deemed to be essential for entry-level competency, this workbook provides only cursory coverage for those chapters.

In order to use this workbook most effectively, students are advised to answer each set of exercises immediately after studying the appropriate anatomic and radiographic sections from *Merrill's Atlas*. Students can check their answers with those provided at the end of each volume. All exercise items are directly referenced to the corresponding information from *Merrill's Atlas*.

ACKNOWLEDGMENTS

My appreciation is extended to those who were instrumental in the development of this workbook. The first, of course, is my wife Sharon. The simple dedication in the front of this workbook does not adequately express my appreciation for all her support and assistance with this publication and with every goal I ever pursued. For more than 30 years she has given me more than I can ever return in kind.

Sometimes not all the difficulties of a major writing project are fully realized by an author when initially accepting the task. The successful completion of many publications is often affected by how much support the author receives from family members. I am fortunate to have the complete support of my family. For that reason I need to recognize my two children who allowed me to temporarily withdraw my presence from their activities. My son, Steven G. Hayes Jr., A.S.R.T., R.T.(R) (ARRT), is very supportive of everything I do, especially with the development of this workbook. Because he is an experienced radiologic educator and technologist, his knowledge of radiographic positioning was very beneficial to me in obtaining some of the radiographic images I needed, and with assisting in the development of the text. I value his support and advice. I also want to thank my daughter, Tonya, for her understanding when I was excusing myself from family activities so I could sustain my production schedule. To both, I apologize for depriving them of my time during the development of this workbook.

Another radiologic educator, Jackie Miller, B.S.R.T., R.T.(R) (ARRT), has been a close friend and colleague of mine longer than either of us can remember. I know no one who has more common sense than Jackie. Other than my wife, he probably knows me better than anyone else does. I appreciate his assistance is obtaining some of the radiographs used in this workbook and the long-term encouragement he has given me in all my endeavors.

I also want to recognize two members of Mosby-Year Book, Inc.: Jeanne Rowland and Lisa Potts. Jeanne is the acquisitions editor who first proposed this workbook project to me. I appreciate the confidence she had in me from the very onset. Lisa, an accomplished developmental editor, was very important in assisting me throughout the entire development of this workbook. She was always available to answer every question I had and provided useful advice that made my work so much easier. Thank you, Lisa.

Last but not least, I want to thank Philip W. Ballinger, M.S., R.T. (R). He was quick to answer my technical questions concerning *Merrill's Atlas* and offered significant suggestions.

I have been lucky to have the love and support of many wonderful people. Those I have just mentioned are the ones who really are responsible for this workbook.

Steven G. Hayes Sr.

TABLE OF CONTENTS

Volume Two

Chapter 14: Mouth and Salivary Glands 1
Chapter 15: Anterior Part of the Neck 11
Chapter 16: Digestive System: Abdomen, Liver, Spleen, and Biliary Tract 19
Chapter 17: Digestive System: Alimentary Tract 41
Chapter 18: Urinary System 79
Chapter 19: Reproductive System 97
Chapter 20: Skull 113
Chapter 21: Facial Bones 155
Chapter 22: Paranasal Sinuses 177
Chapter 23: Temporal Bone 189
Chapter 24: Mammography 195
Chapter 25: Central Nervous System 203
Chapter 26: Circulatory System 213
Chapter 27: Sectional Anatomy for Radiographers 235
Appendix: Supplemental Exercises for Skull Positioning 261
Answers to Exercises
Chapter 14 283
Chapter 15 283
Chapter 16 284
Chapter 17 287
Chapter 18 291
Chapter 19 293
Chapter 20 294
Chapter 21 299
Chapter 22 301
Chapter 23 302
Chapter 24 303
Chapter 25 304
Chapter 26 305
Chapter 27 307
Answers to Appendix 309

Chapter 14
MOUTH AND SALIVARY GLANDS

Chapter 14 Review

Instructions: This exercise provides an anatomic review of the mouth and salivary glands and a cursory review of sialography. Items require you to identify structures, fill in missing words, provide a short answer, match columns, or choose true or false. Explain any statement you believe is false.

1. Identify each lettered structure in Figure 14-1.

A. _____

B. _____

C. _____

D. _____

E. _____

F. _____

G. _____

H. _____

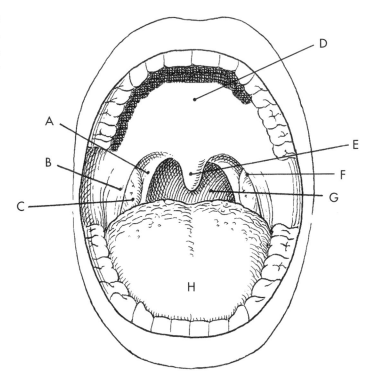

Fig. 14-1. Anterior aspect of oral cavity.

2. Identify each lettered structure in Figure 14-2.

A. _____

B. _____

C. _____

D. _____

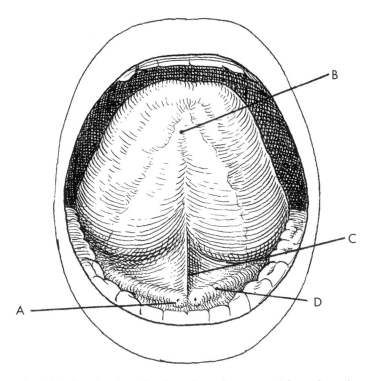

Fig. 14-2. Anterior view of undersurface of tongue and floor of mouth.

3. Identify each lettered structure in Figure 14-3.

A. _____

B. _____

C. _____

D. _____

E. _____

F. _____

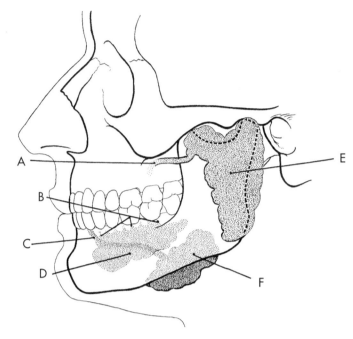

Fig. 14-3. Salivary glands from left lateral aspect.

4. Identify each lettered structure in Figure 14-4.

A. _____

B. _____

C. _____

D. _____

E. _____

F. _____

G. _____

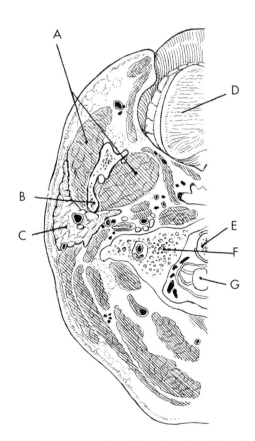

Fig. 14-4. Transverse section of face showing relation of parotid gland to mandibular ramus. (Auricle not shown in illustration.)

5. Identify each lettered structure in Figure 14-5.

A. _____

B. _____

C. _____

D. _____

E. _____

F. _____

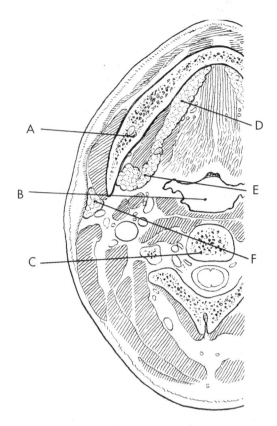

Fig. 14-5. Transverse section of face showing relation of submandibular (submaxillary) and sublingual glands to surrounding structures. (Auricle not shown in illustration.)

6. What is the first division of the digestive system?

7. Define *mastication.*

8. What structures serve the function of mastication?

9. What is the purpose of saliva?

10. Name the three pairs of salivary glands.

11. Match the glands in Column A with the ducts in Column B.

Column A

   ___ 1. parotid gland

   ___ 2. sublingual gland

   ___ 3. submandibular gland

Column B

a. Wharton's duct

b. Stensen's duct

c. ducts of Rivinus

12. The main duct of Rivinus is also called _____ duct.

13. What gland does Bartholin's duct help drain?

14. Define *sialography.*

15. What two imaging modalities have greatly reduced the frequency of sialography?

16. What type of contrast medium is used for sialography?

17. Why can only one salivary gland at a time be examined by the sialographic method?

18. List two reasons that preliminary radiographs are made before the introduction of the contrast medium.

19. Why should the patient be given a secretory stimulant?

20. Name the three projections that demonstrate the salivary glands and ducts.

21. The tangential projection is made to demonstrate the _____ gland.

22. What sialographic projection demonstrates either the parotid glands or the submandibular glands?

23. True or False. The patient may be positioned prone or supine for the tangential projection.

24. True or False. The mandibular ramus should be parallel with the plane of the film for the tangential projection.

25. True or False. Parotid glands on both sides of the face can be demonstrated with the same tangential exposure.

26. What salivary gland can be demonstrated with a lateral projection when the patient's head is adjusted so that the median sagittal plane is rotated approximately 15 degrees toward the cassette from true lateral and the central ray is directed to a point 1 inch (2.5 cm) above the mandibular ramus?

27. What salivary gland can be demonstrated with a lateral projection when the patient's head is positioned true lateral and a perpendicular central ray is directed to the inferior margin of the mandibular angle?

28. For the lateral projection to demonstrate the submandibular gland, what is the purpose of pressing the tongue to the floor of the mouth?

29. What salivary glands are demonstrated with the axial projection (intraoral method)?

30. What sialographic projection is the only projection that demonstrates an unobstructed image of the sublingual gland area?

31. What sialographic image can be made with occlusal film?

32. What sialographic projection directs the central ray along the lateral surface of the mandibular ramus?

33. Examine Figure 14-6 and answer the questions that follow.

    a. What projection does this image represent?

    b. What salivary gland is demonstrated?

    c. What special breathing technique can be performed by the patient to improve the radiographic demonstration of the gland with this projection?

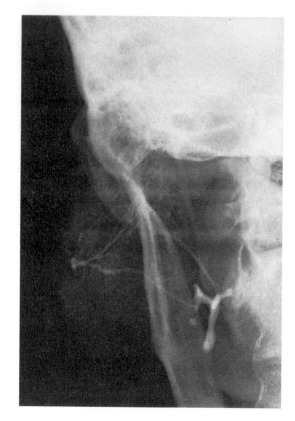

Fig. 14-6. Sialogram showing opacification of a gland.

34. Examine Figure 14-7 and answer the questions that follow.

    a. What projection does this image represent?

    b. What salivary gland is demonstrated?

    c. To what duct does the arrow point?

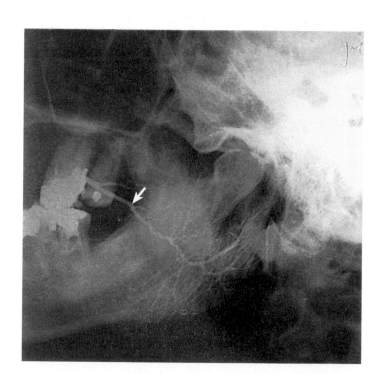

Fig. 14-7. Sialogram showing opacification of a gland.

35. Examine Figure 14-8 and answer the questions that follow.

   a. What projection does this image represent?

   b. What salivary gland is demonstrated?

   c. To what duct does the arrow point?

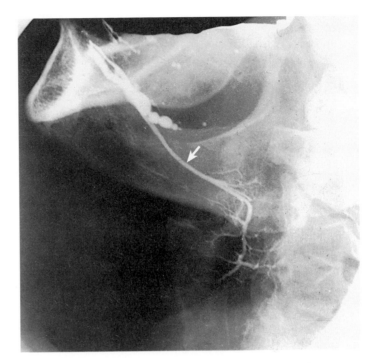

Fig. 14-8. Sialogram showing opacification of a gland.

Self-Test: Mouth and Salivary Glands

Instructions: Answer the following questions by selecting the best choice.

1. What is the first division of the digestive system?

   a. mouth
   b. stomach
   c. salivary glands
   d. small intestine

2. Which salivary gland is the largest?

   a. parotid
   b. sublingual
   c. submandibular

3. Which salivary gland is drained by Wharton's duct?

   a. parotid
   b. sublingual
   c. submandibular

4. What other term refers to the parotid duct?

   a. Stensen's duct
   b. Wharton's duct
   c. Bartholin's duct

5. Which salivary gland is located along the lateral aspect of the mandibular ramus?

   a. parotid
   b. sublingual
   c. submandibular

6. For sialography, into which structure is the contrast medium injected?

   a. vein
   b. artery
   c. muscle
   d. salivary duct

7. Which sialographic projection directs the central ray along the mandibular ramus?

   a. axial
   b. lateral
   c. tangential
   d. verticosubmental

8. Which sialographic projection demonstrates a parotid gland superimposed over a mandibular ramus?

   a. axial
   b. lateral
   c. tangential
   d. verticosubmental

9. Which two sialographic projections best demonstrate the parotid gland?

   a. axial and lateral
   b. axial and verticosubmental
   c. tangential and lateral
   d. tangential and verticosubmental

10. Which sialographic projection demonstrates an unobstructed view of the sublingual area?

    a. axial
    b. lateral
    c. tangential
    d. verticosubmental

If your school has access to Mosby's Radiographic Instructional Series on Anatomy, Positioning, and Procedures, review Unit 14 at this time; your instructor may request that you respond to the series' exercises on paper. This unit covers the following examinations:

Sialography
Parotid gland
Parotid and submandibular glands
Submandibular and sublingual glands

Chapter 15
ANTERIOR PART OF THE NECK

Chapter 15 Review

Instructions: This exercise is a review of the anatomy and radiography of the anterior part of the neck. Items require you to identify structues, fill in missing words, or provide a short answer.

1. Identify each lettered structure in Figure 15-1.

A. _____

B. _____

C. _____

D. _____

E. _____

F. _____

G. _____

H. _____

I. _____

J. _____

K. _____

L. _____

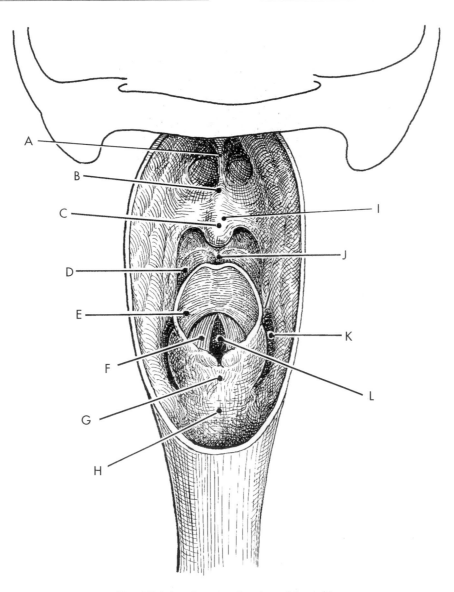

Fig. 15-1. Interior posterior view of the neck.

2. Identify each lettered structure in Figure 15-2.

A. _____   H. _____

B. _____   I. _____

C. _____   J. _____

D. _____   K. _____

E. _____   L. _____

F. _____   M. _____

G. _____   N. _____

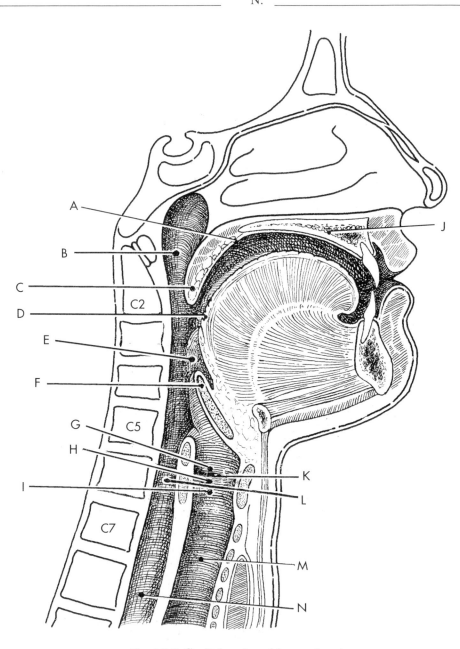

Fig. 15-2. Sagittal section of face and neck.

3. Identify each lettered structure in Figure 15-3.

A. _____

B. _____

C. _____

D. _____

E. _____

F. _____

G. _____

H. _____

I. _____

J. _____

K. _____

L. _____

M. _____

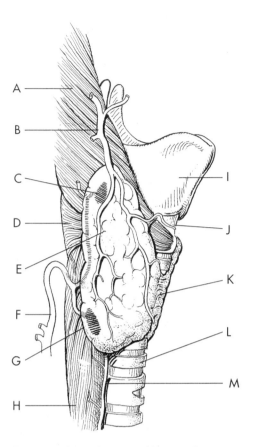

Fig. 15-3. Lateral aspect of laryngeal area.

4. Identify each lettered structure in Figure 15-4.

A. _____

B. _____

C. _____

D. _____

E. _____

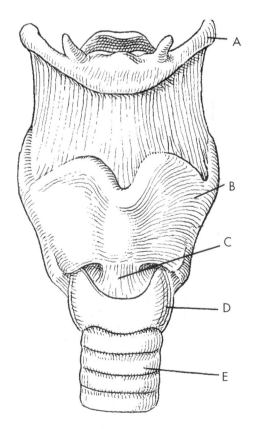

Fig. 15-4. Anterior aspect of larynx.

5. Identify each lettered structure in Figure 15-5.

A. _____   F. _____

B. _____   G. _____

C. _____   H. _____

D. _____   I. _____

E. _____

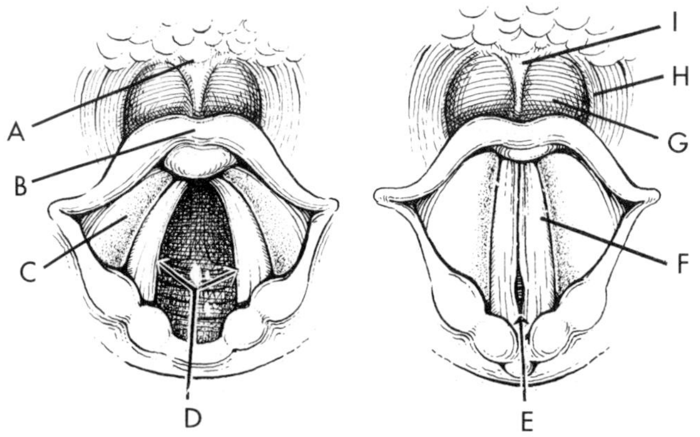

Fig. 15-5. Superior aspect of larynx (open and closed true vocal folds).

6. For radiographic purposes, the neck is divided into _____ and _____ portions.

7. The upper part of the respiratory system located in the anterior part of the neck is the _____.

8. The upper part of the digestive system located in the anterior part of the neck is the _____.

9. The two major glands located in the anterior part of the neck are the _____ gland and _____ gland.

10. What structure of the upper neck serves as a passage for both food and air and is common to the respiratory and digestive systems?

11. The portion of the pharynx located above the soft palate is the _____.

12. The portion of the pharynx located from the soft palate to the hyoid bone is the _____.

13. The organ of voice is the _____.

14. The structure that comprises the vocal apparatus of the larynx is the _____.

15. The projections that demonstrate the pharynx and larynx are the _____ and _____ projections.

16. During what four bodily functions are radiographs of the pharynx and larynx made?

17. Identify the body position in which the patient should be placed for each of the following examinations of the pharynx and larynx:

    a. Tomographic studies: _____

    b. AP and lateral projections: _____

18. For the AP projection, the central ray should be directed perpendicularly to the _____

    _____.

19. Identify the x-ray tube and film centering points for the lateral projection of the following structures:

    a. Nasopharynx: _____

    b. Oropharynx: _____

    c. Larynx: _____

20. Identify each lettered structure in Figure 15-6.

A. _____   C. _____

B. _____   D. _____

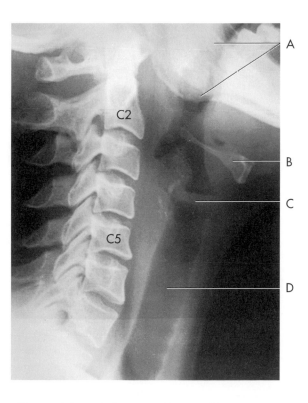

Fig. 15-6. Lateral pharynx and larynx. Valsalva maneuver.

Self-Test: Anterior Part of the Neck

Instructions: Answer the following questions by selecting the best choice.

1. What is the musculomembranous structure located in front of the vertebrae and behind the nose, the mouth, and the larynx?

   a. pharynx
   b. trachea
   c. glottis
   d. esophagus

2. Which structure of the neck consists of various cartilages, including the epiglottis, the thyroid, and the cricoid cartilages?

   a. larynx
   b. pharynx
   c. trachea
   d. esophagus

3. Which structure forms the laryngeal prominence?

   a. epiglottis
   b. true vocal folds
   c. thyroid cartilage
   d. cricoid cartilage

4. Which structure prevents leakage into the larynx during swallowing?

   a. pharynx
   b. epiglottis
   c. cricoid cartilage
   d. thyroid cartilage

5. What is the most superiorly located structure of the neck?

   a. larynx
   b. pharynx
   c. glottis
   d. epiglottis

6. For the AP projection to demonstrate the pharynx and larynx, to which level of the patient should the central ray be directed?

   a. C1
   b. C7
   c. mandibular angles
   d. laryngeal prominence

7. For the preliminary AP and lateral projections to demonstrate the pharynx and larynx, when should the exposures be made to ensure filling the throat passages with air?

   a. after suspended inhalation
   b. after suspended exhalation
   c. during inhalation
   d. during exhalation

8. Which body position should be used for tomographic examinations of the pharynx and larynx?

   a. prone
   b. supine
   c. upright lateral
   d. recumbent lateral

9. For the lateral projection to demonstrate the oropharynx, to which level of the patient should the central ray be directed?

   a. external acoustic meatuses
   b. mandibular angles
   c. laryngeal prominence
   d. C7

10. Which procedure should be performed by the patient for tomographic studies of pharyngolaryngeal structures?

    a. quiet inhalation through the nose
    b. phonation of a high-pitched "e-e-e"
    c. suspended respiration after inhalation
    d. suspended respiration after exhalation

If your school has access to Mosby's Radiographic Instructional Series on Anatomy, Positioning, and Procedures, review Unit 15 at this time; your instructor may request that you respond to the series' exercises on paper. This unit covers the following examinations:

Soft palate, pharynx, and larynx: Alternative examination methods
   Palatography
   Nasopharyngography
   Pharyngography
   Laryngopharyngography
   Tomolaryngography
   Positive-contrast laryngopharyngography
Thyroid gland
Pharynx and larynx
Soft palate, pharynx, and larynx: Radiographic examination

Chapter 16
THE DIGESTIVE SYSTEM: ABDOMEN, LIVER, SPLEEN, AND BILIARY TRACT

Part 1

ANATOMY OF THE ABDOMEN, THE LIVER, THE SPLEEN, AND THE BILIARY TRACT

Exercise 1

Instructions: This exercise pertains to the abdominal contents. Items require you to identify structures.

1. Identify each lettered structure in Figure 16-1.

A. _____   J. _____

B. _____   K. _____

C. _____   L. _____

D. _____   M. _____

E. _____   N. _____

F. _____   O. _____

G. _____   P. _____

H. _____   Q. _____

I. _____   R. _____

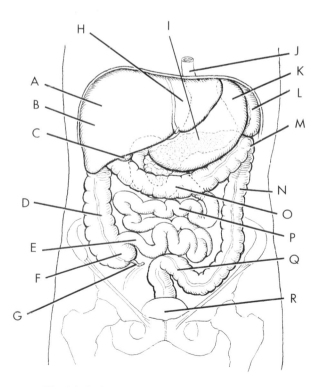

Fig. 16-1. Anterior aspect of abdominal viscera.

2. Identify each lettered structure in Figure 16-2.

A. _____   I. _____

B. _____   J. _____

C. _____   K. _____

D. _____   L. _____

E. _____   M. _____

F. _____   N. _____

G. _____   O. _____

H. _____

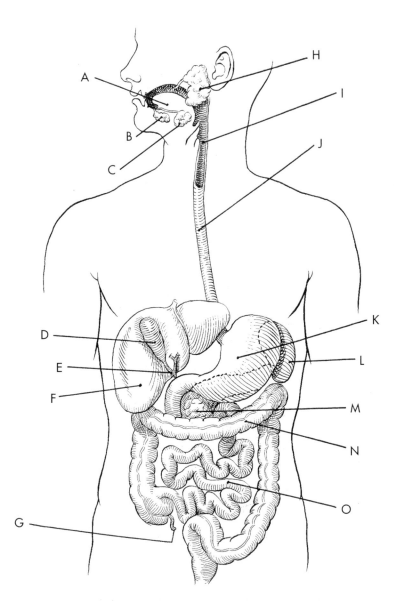

Fig. 16-2. Alimentary tract and its accessory organs.

3. Identify each lettered structure in Figure 16-3.

A. _____

B. _____

C. _____

D. _____

E. _____

F. _____

G. _____

H. _____

I. _____

J. _____

K. _____

L. _____

M. _____

N. _____

O. _____

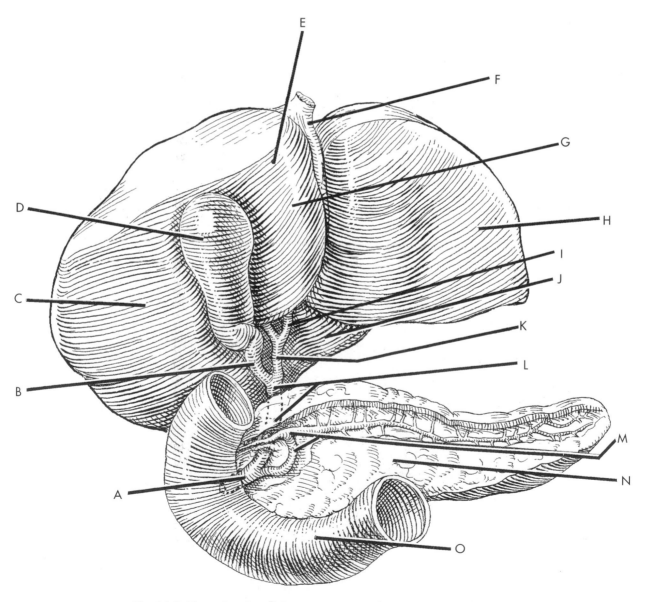

Fig. 16-3. Visceral surface (inferoposterior aspect) of liver and gall bladder.

4. Identify each lettered structure in Figure 16-4.

A. _____   F. _____

B. _____   G. _____

C. _____   H. _____

D. _____   I. _____

E. _____   J. _____

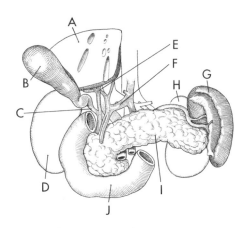

Fig. 16-4. Visceral (inferoposterior) surface of gall bladder and bile ducts.

5. Identify each lettered structure in Figure 16-5.

A. _____   E. _____

B. _____   F. _____

C. _____   G. _____

D. _____

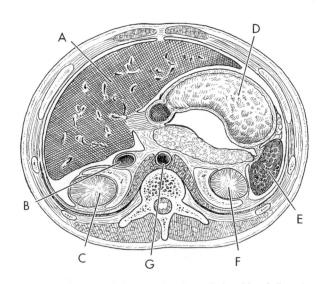

Fig. 16-5. Sectional image of upper abdomen showing relationship of digestive system components.

Exercise 2

Instructions: This exercise pertains to the liver, the biliary system, the pancreas, and the spleen. Items require you to fill in missing words, provide a short answer, or choose true or false. Explain any statement you believe is false.

1. The name of the double-walled seromembranous sac that lines the abdominal cavity is the _____.

2. List the names of the two layers of the peritoneum.

3. The outer layer of the peritoneum that contacts the underside of the diaphragm is called the _____ layer.

4. The inner layer of the peritoneum that contacts various organs is called the _____ layer.

5. What organ occupies most of the right hypochondrium and the epigastrium regions of the abdomen?

6. The largest organ in the abdominal cavity is the _____.

7. The radiographically significant physiologic function of the liver is the production of _____.

8. The right and left hepatic ducts join to form the _____ _____ _____.

9. The cystic duct enables bile from the liver to be stored in the _____ _____.

10. The gall bladder is usually located on the inferior side of the right lobe of the _____.

11. **True or False. In a hypersthenic patient, the gall bladder is situated high and well away from the median sagittal plane.**

12. True or False. The gall bladder is located posterior to the liver in the retroperitoneal space.

13. The common hepatic duct unites with the cystic duct to form the _____ _____ _____.

14. In 20% of subjects, before entering the duodenum, the common bile duct joins with the _____ _____.

15. The muscular contraction of the gall bladder is activated by a hormone called _____.

16. Another name for the ampulla of Vater is _____ _____.

17. The gland that produces insulin is the _____.

18. True or False. The pancreas cannot be demonstrated with plain radiography.

19. True or False. The spleen is an organ of the lymphatic system.

20. True or False. The pancreas and the liver secrete specialized digestive juices into the small intestine.

—————— Part 2

POSITIONING OF THE ABDOMEN AND GALL BLADDER

Exercise 1 Positioning for the Abdomen

Instructions: A variety of radiographic procedures are used to demonstrate the abdomen and its contents. A patient is usually first examined with plain radiography before specialized studies using contrast media are performed. This exercise reviews the positions and projections commonly used to produce radiographs of the abdomen without the introduction of a contrast medium. Items require you to fill in missing words, provide a short answer, or choose true or false. Explain any statement you believe is false.

Items 1 through 15 pertain to the AP and PA projections.

1. What commonly used acronym refers to the AP projection of the abdomen with the patient supine?

2. For the AP projection with the patient supine, at what level of the patient should the cassette be placed?

3. List the two levels of the patient to which the cassette should be centered when the patient is positioned upright, and give the reason for the difference in cassette placement.

4. List the three considerations for the use of gonadal shielding in abdominal radiography.

5. The kilovoltage peak for the sthenic patient should be approximately _____ kVp.

6. Respiration should be suspended after _____. Explain why.

7. Explain why the exposure should not be made for 1 or 2 seconds after respiration is suspended.

8. True or False. A perpendicular central ray should be directed to the center of the cassette.

9. List three evaluation criteria that can be used when examining a KUB radiograph to determine whether the patient was rotated.

10. What structure of the upper abdomen should be seen on the radiograph when the patient is upright? Explain why.

11. What two identification markers should be seen on the radiograph when the patient is upright?

12. With reference to radiation protection, what is the advantage of the PA projection over the AP projection?

13. What three projections usually comprise the three-way or acute abdomen series?

14. Why is a chest radiograph included as part of the acute abdomen series?

15. In the acute abdomen series, what radiograph should be substituted for the upright abdomen radiograph when the patient is unable to stand?

Items 16 through 26 pertain to the lateral decubitus positions.

16. What is the advantage of a lateral decubitus position over the KUB?

17. Why is the left lateral decubitus position preferred when the patient is unable to stand for the upright abdomen?

18. Describe the position of the patient for the left lateral decubitus position.

19. With reference to the patient, describe the placement and centering of the cassette.

20. What breathing instructions should be given to the patient?

21. Describe how and to where the central ray should be directed.

22. What side of the abdomen should be demonstrated if only one side can be imaged and the patient may have free air in the abdomen?

23. What side of the abdomen should be demonstrated if only one side can be imaged and the patient is suspected to have fluid levels within the abdominal cavity?

24. What structure of the upper abdomen should be demonstrated on the radiograph?

25. What identification markers should be seen on the radiograph?

26. Examine Figure 16-6 and state the complete name of the projection for which the patient is positioned.

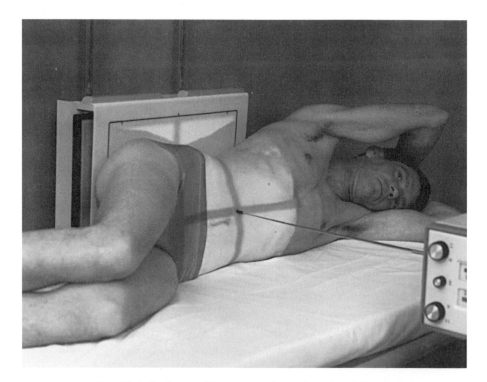

Fig. 16-6. Patient positioned for radiograph of the abdomen.

Items 27 through 33 pertain to the lateral projection.

27. True or False. A lateral projection of the abdomen can be performed with the patient placed in either the right lateral recumbent position or the left lateral recumbent position.

28. True or False. The exposure should be made after the patient has suspended respiration after full inhalation.

29. To what level of the patient should the cassette be centered?

30. If a compression band is needed to immobilize the patient, where should it be placed?

31. Where exactly should the central ray enter the patient?

32. What two areas of the image can be closely examined to determine whether the patient was rotated?

33. Examine Figure 16-7 and state the complete name of the position the patient is in.

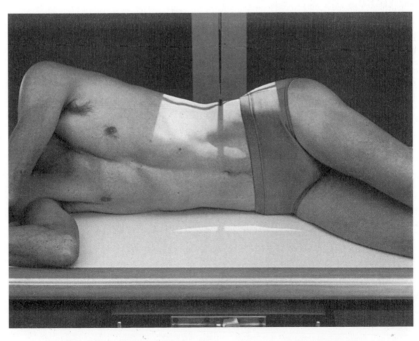

Fig. 16-7. Patient positioned for radiograph of the abdomen.

Items 34 through 40 pertain to the lateral position with the patient in the dorsal decubitus position.

34. What is the name of the radiographic position that produces a lateral image of the abdomen with the patient in the supine position?

35. To what level of the patient should the long axis of the film be centered?

36. How far above the level of the iliac crests should the central ray enter the patient?

37. What purpose is served by having the patient slightly flex the knees?

38. The exposure should be made after _____.

39. True or False. The central ray should be horizontally directed to the center of the film.

40. List the three evaluation criteria that indicates the patient was properly positioned for the lateral projection (dorsal decubitus position).

Exercise 2 Contrast Studies for the Gall Bladder

Instructions: This exercise pertains to the radiographic demonstration of the gall bladder with a contrast medium. Items require you to fill in missing words, provide a short answer, or choose true or false. Explain any statement you believe is false.

1. The radiographic visualization of the gall bladder after introduction of a contrast medium is termed _____.

2. The most common method by which a contrast medium is introduced into a patient for cholecystography is the

   _____ method.

3. Two common abbreviations for oral cholecystography are _____ and _____.

4. An oral cholecystopaque is absorbed through the intestines and transported to the liver by the _____ vein.

5. List important information that can be learned about each of the following structures with OCG:

   a. Liver: _____

   b. Biliary ducts: _____

   c. Gall bladder: _____

6. The most common pathologic reason for performing OCG is to demonstrate _____.

7. **True or False.** Pure cholesterol gallstones appear as negative filling defects within the opacified bile.

8. **True or False.** Gallstones containing calcium can often be seen on plain radiography before the introduction of a contrast medium.

9. List six topics that should be included in written instructions given to the patient preparing for OCG.

10. After the OCG patient arrives in the radiography department for the examination, why is it important to determine whether the patient experienced vomiting or diarrhea after ingesting the oral cholecystopaque tablets?

11. Why should OCG patients be scheduled for examinations in the early part of the morning?

12. What two purposes may be served by performing a general survey scout radiograph of the patient prior to preparation for OCG?

13. If the use of a laxative is part of the preparation for OCG, why should the patient be instructed to not use a laxative less than 24 hours before swallowing the oral cholecystopaque tablets?

14. After consuming the oral cholecystopaque tablets but before arriving in the radiography department for the scheduled OCG, the patient is allowed what food or drink?

15. What imaging modality is often used to complement OCG if gall bladder films fail to provide a diagnosis?

Items 16 through 31 pertain to the PA projection.

16. True or False. The PA projection can be performed with the patient either in the prone position or upright.

17. True or False. The left side of the patient should be centered to the midline of the table.

18. Which focal spot size—large or small—should be used for radiography of the gall bladder?

19. What maximum exposure time should be used for exposing the cassettes?

20. What procedure should be performed to prevent pendulous breasts of female patients from superimposing the gall bladder?

21. With the patient prone, why should the left cheek rather than the right cheek rest on a pillow?

22. What can be done to the lower limbs to relieve pressure on the toes when the patient is prone?

23. The exposure should be made after the patient has suspended respiration after _____.

24. How many seconds should elapse after the patient suspends respiration before the exposure is made? Explain why.

25. Examine the radiographs in Figures 16-8 and 16-9 and answer the questions that follow.

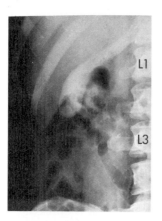

Fig. 16-8. Gall bladder radiograph.

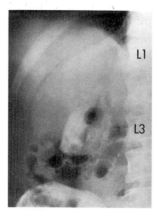

Fig. 16-9. Gall bladder radiograph.

a. Which radiograph was exposed after the patient suspended respiration after exhalation?

b. Which radiograph should be marked to indicate the specific phase of respiration when the exposure was made?

26. What procedure should be performed for a subsequent PA projection radiograph with the patient prone if the first PA projection radiograph demonstrates the gall bladder superimposed with rib shadows?

27. Identify the body habitus type (sthenic, asthenic, or hypersthenic) for which each of the following central ray centering levels is used:

    a. 9th costal cartilage: _____

    b. 2 inches (5 cm) above the 9th costal cartilage: _____

    c. 2 inches (5 cm) below the 9th costal cartilage: _____

28. Is the centering point for the patient who is moved to the standing position from the prone position somewhat higher or lower?

29. How many inches does the gall bladder's position shift when the prone patient is placed in the upright position?

30. When the patient is positioned in the upright position, gallstones that are heavier than bile should be demonstrated in the

    _____ portion of the gall bladder.

31. Listed below are statements pertaining to the prone and upright positions. In the space provided, write **P** if the statement pertains to the prone position or **U** if the statement pertains to the upright position.

    ____ a. produces an irregularly circular or triangular image of the gall bladder

    ____ b. produces a foreshortened image of the gall bladder

    ____ c. is best to show mobility of the gall bladder

    ____ d. is best to show many gallstones that are too small to be seen individually

    ____ e. generally requires higher localization centering than the other PA projection

    ____ f. can show different layers of gallstones

    ____ g. usually projects an image of a more vertical gall bladder

    ____ h. radiograph should be marked to indicate the position of the patient

Items 32 **through 42 pertain** to the left anterior oblique (LAO) position and the right lateral projection.

32. **The LAO position is** particularly effective in separating the shadow of the gall bladder from the _____

    _____.

33. How many degrees should the patient be rotated from the prone position for the LAO projection?

34. List three factors that affect the degree of rotation when positioning the patient for the LAO projection.

35. Who requires more rotation, thin patients or large patients?

36. Why should the recumbent patient be positioned LAO instead of RPO even though both positions produce similar images?

37. Why should a radiolucent foam wedge be placed against the anterior surface of the abdomen when the recumbent patient is placed in the LAO position?

38. Why is the right lateral position preferred over the left lateral position when the lateral projection is performed?

39. The right lateral projection is sometimes used to differentiate gallstones from _____ stones.

40. The exposure should be made after the patient has suspended respiration after _____.

41. For whom is the right lateral position useful for separating the shadows of the gall bladder and the vertebrae, exceptionally large or exceptionally thin patients?

42. Cholecystograms should demonstrate the gall bladder and surrounding structures in a _____ scale of contrast.

Items 43 through 45 pertain to the right lateral decubitus position.

43. True or False. The right lateral decubitus position is used for stratification studies of the low-placed gall bladder.

44. True or False. The left lateral decubitus position should be performed if the patient is unable to stand or to be positioned for the right lateral decubitus position.

45. Examine the images of gall bladders in Figures 16-10 through 16-13. Based on the appearance or the location of each gall bladder in relationship to its surrounding structures, identify the most likely position in which the patient was placed for the exposure: PA (prone), PA (upright), left anterior oblique, or right lateral decubitus.

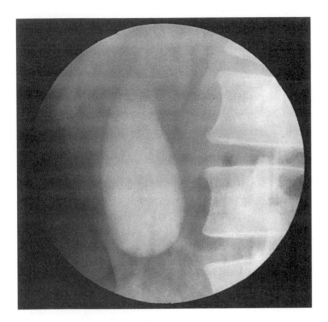

Fig. 16-10. A radiograph of a gall bladder.

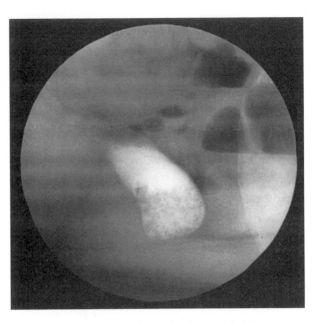

Fig. 16-11. A radiograph of a gall bladder.

a. Figure 16-10: _____

b. Figure 16-11: _____

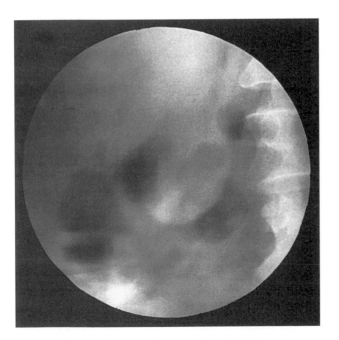

Fig. 16-12. A radiograph of a gall bladder.

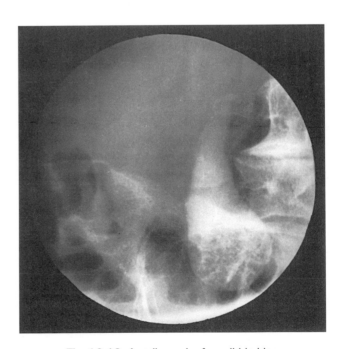

Fig. 16-13. A radiograph of a gall bladder.

c. Figure 16-12: _____

d. Figure 16-13: _____

Self-Test: The Abdomen and the Gall Bladder

Instructions: Answer the following questions by selecting the best choice.

1. Which organ produces bile?

   a. liver
   b. spleen
   c. pancreas
   d. gall bladder

2. Which body function is performed by the pancreas?

   a. filters blood
   b. produces bile
   c. produces lymphocytes
   d. produces digestive juices

3. Which organ serves to store and concentrate bile?

   a. liver
   b. spleen
   c. pancreas
   d. gall bladder

4. The muscular contraction of the gall bladder is activated by:

   a. bile.
   b. cholecystokinin.
   c. pancreatic juices.
   d. cholecystolithiasis.

5. The spleen is part of which body system?

   a. urinary
   b. digestive
   c. lymphatic
   d. endocrine

6. In which organ are the islets of Langerhans found?

   a. liver
   b. spleen
   c. pancreas
   d. gall bladder

7. How many major lobes does the liver have?

   a. 1
   b. 2
   c. 3
   d. 4

8. The mesentery and omenta folds are formed by the:

   a. liver.
   b. pancreas.
   c. peritoneum.
   d. gall bladder.

9. Which organ is supplied blood by the portal vein?

   a. liver
   b. spleen
   c. pancreas
   d. gall bladder

10. Which duct is formed by the merging of the right and left hepatic ducts?

    a. cystic
    b. pancreatic
    c. common bile
    d. common hepatic

11. Which duct is formed by the union of the cystic duct with the common hepatic duct?

    a. pancreatic
    b. common bile
    c. left hepatic
    d. right hepatic

12. Where do the pancreatic and common bile ducts terminate?

    a. ileum
    b. duodenum
    c. gall bladder
    d. large intestine

13. Which duct connects the gall bladder to the common hepatic duct?

    a. cystic
    b. pancreatic
    c. common bile
    d. right hepatic

14. Which three projections/positions usually comprise the acute abdomen series?

    a. KUB, AP upright abdomen, and PA chest
    b. KUB, right lateral decubitus abdomen, and PA chest
    c. left lateral decubitus abdomen, dorsal decubitus abdomen, and PA chest
    d. right lateral decubitus abdomen, left lateral decubitus abdomen, and dorsal decubitus abdomen

15. To which level of the patient should the cassette be centered for the KUB?

    a. T10 vertebral body
    b. L3 vertebral body
    c. 2 inches (5 cm) above the iliac crests
    d. the iliac crests

16. For the AP upright abdomen radiograph of an adult of average size, why should the cassette be slightly raised above the centering level used for the KUB radiograph?

    a. to include the bladder
    b. to include the diaphragm
    c. to visualize gallstones
    d. to visualize kidney stones

17. For the KUB radiograph, when should respiration be suspended, and what effect will that have on the patient?

    a. on full inhalation; depress the diaphragm
    b. on full inhalation; elevate the diaphragm
    c. on full exhalation; depress the diaphragm
    d. on full exhalation; elevate the diaphragm

18. Why is it desirable to include the diaphragm in the upright abdomen radiograph?

    a. to demonstrate free air in the abdomen
    b. to demonstrate fluid levels in the thorax
    c. to demonstrate fluid levels in the abdomen
    d. to demonstrate calculi in the gall bladder and kidneys

19. Which guideline is not necessary to follow when deciding whether to use gonadal shielding for the KUB radiograph?

    a. Patient has reasonable reproductive potential.
    b. Purpose for doing the examination is not compromised.
    c. Gonads lie within 2 inches (5 cm) of the primary beam.
    d. Permission to use gonadal shielding is granted by the patient.

20. Which position should be used to demonstrate free air within the abdominal cavity when the patient is unable to stand for the upright abdomen radiograph?

    a. KUB
    b. dorsal decubitus abdomen
    c. left lateral decubitus abdomen
    d. right lateral decubitus abdomen

21. Which position does not demonstrate free air levels within the abdomen?

    a. KUB (supine)
    b. upright
    c. dorsal decubitus
    d. left lateral decubitus

22. The major advantage that the PA projection of the abdomen has over the AP projection of the abdomen is that the PA projection:

    a. reduces the OID (OFD) of the kidneys.
    b. reduces the exposure dose to the gonads.
    c. magnifies gallstones for better visualization.
    d. projects the pubic rami below the urinary bladder.

23. Which position of the abdomen requires the patient lateral recumbent on the left side and the central ray directed along the median sagittal plane, entering the anterior surface of the patient's abdomen at the level of the iliac crests?

    a. dorsal decubitus
    b. ventral decubitus
    c. left lateral decubitus
    d. right lateral decubitus

24. Which position of the abdomen requires the patient supine and the central ray directed to a lateral side of the patient, entering slightly anterior to the median coronal plane?

    a. dorsal decubitus
    b. ventral decubitus
    c. left lateral decubitus
    d. right lateral decubitus

25. Which projection of the abdomen requires the patient lateral recumbent on the left side, the cassette placed under the patient and centered to the abdomen at the level of the iliac crests, and the central ray directed to enter the right side of the patient slightly anterior to the median coronal plane?

    a. left lateral
    b. right lateral
    c. left lateral decubitus
    d. right lateral decubitus

26. The dorsal decubitus, the left lateral, and the left lateral decubitus positions of the abdomen all require:

    a. the patient to suspend respiration after exhalation.
    b. the patient to suspend respiration after inhalation.
    c. the central ray to enter the left side of the patient.
    d. the central ray to enter the anterior side of the abdomen.

27. For the dorsal decubitus position of the abdomen, where should the central ray enter the patient?

    a. 2 inches (5 cm) anterior to the median coronal plane at the level of the iliac crests
    b. 2 inches (5 cm) anterior to the median coronal plane and 2 inches above the level of the iliac crests
    c. 2 inches (5 cm) posterior to the median coronal plane at the level of the iliac crests
    d. 2 inches (5 cm) posterior to the median coronal plane and 2 inches above the level of the iliac crests

28. For the dorsal decubitus position of the abdomen, which procedure should be performed to ensure that the entire abdomen is included on the radiograph?

    a. Use support cushions to elevate the patient.
    b. Direct the central ray to a point 2 inches (5 cm) below the iliac crests.
    c. Center the cassette to the level of the xiphoid process.
    d. Center the cassette to the anterior surface of the abdomen.

29. Which structures should be examined to see whether the patient was rotated for the lateral projection of the abdomen?

    a. pelvis and lumbar vertebrae
    b. pelvis and thoracic vertebrae
    c. diaphragm and lumbar vertebrae
    d. diaphragm and thoracic vertebrae

30. Which imaging procedure should be part of the OCG examination?

    a. Use long exposure times and long scale of contrast.
    b. Use long exposure times and short scale of contrast.
    c. Use short exposure times and long scale of contrast.
    d. Use short exposure times and short scale of contrast.

31. For oral cholecystography procedures, when should respiration be suspended, and what effect will that have on the position of the gall bladder?

    a. on full inhalation; depress the gall bladder
    b. on full inhalation; elevate the gall bladder
    c. on full exhalation; depress the gall bladder
    d. on full exhalation; elevate the gall bladder

32. Which procedure should be performed when the OCG patient is rotated from a prone position to the left anterior oblique position?

    a. Make the exposure after full inhalation.
    b. Center the cassette to the level of the diaphragm.
    c. Center the cassette to the left side of the patient.
    d. Place a radiolucent foam wedge under the abdomen.

33. For the OCG examination of the patient of average build, where should the cassette be centered?

    a. at the level of the 9th rib on the left side
    b. at the level of the 9th rib on the right side
    c. at the level of the 12th rib on the left side
    d. at the level of the 12th rib on the right side

34. Compared with cassette placement for the patient of average build, for the OCG examination of the hypersthenic patient, the cassette should be moved:

    a. lower.
    b. higher.
    c. to the left of the vertebral column.
    d. more to the lateral side of the right side of the abdomen.

35. Which procedure should be performed for a subsequent PA projection radiograph when the initial PA projection radiograph demonstrated the shadow of the gall bladder superimposed by ribs?

    a. Place the patient in the Trendelenburg position.
    b. Use radiolucent cushions to elevate the patient.
    c. Direct the central ray caudally 10 to 15 degrees.
    d. Make the exposure after full inhalation.

36. Which procedure most effectively separates the shadows of the gall bladder and vertebrae?

    a. Rotate the patient into an oblique position.
    b. Make the exposure after full inhalation.
    c. Place the patient in the Trendelenburg position.
    d. Position the patient for the dorsal decubitus position.

37. Which projection/position best demonstrates the stratification of gallstones?

    a. KUB
    b. right lateral decubitus
    c. RAO with the patient recumbent
    d. PA with the patient prone

38. Which procedure best demonstrates a gall bladder that is situated in the iliac fossa?

    a. Use the prone position.
    b. Use the supine position.
    c. Use the upright position.
    d. Make the exposure after full inhalation.

39. Why should OCG patients be scheduled for early morning appointments?

    a. Prolonged fasting causes the formation of gas.
    b. Scheduling conflicts with fluoroscopy are prevented.
    c. A gall bladder can store contrast medium for only 8 hours.
    d. Continual production of bile dilutes the contrast medium.

40. Which projection/position places the gall bladder closest to the cassette?

    a. PA
    b. KUB
    c. upright LAO
    d. recumbent LPO

41. Which procedure should not be performed as part of patient preparation for the OCG examination?

    a. Administer a cleansing enema to prepare the intestinal tract.
    b. Have the patient take laxatives within 24 hours before swallowing oral contrast medium.
    c. Allow the patient to consume only water after swallowing oral contrast medium.
    d. Give the patient a fat-free evening meal to consume shortly before swallowing oral contrast medium.

42. Which diagnostic modality is most often used when OCG does not adequately demonstrate a gall bladder?

    a. sonography
    b. nuclear medicine
    c. computed tomography
    d. magnetic resonance imaging

43. Which projection produces a foreshortened image of the gall bladder?

    a. right lateral
    b. PA with the patient prone
    c. PA with the patient upright
    d. LAO with the patient upright

44. All of the following gall bladder projections/positions increase the separation of the gall bladder shadow from the vertebrae except the:

    a. PA.
    b. upright LAO.
    c recumbent LAO.
    d. right lateral decubitus.

45. Which procedure should be performed for the left PA oblique projection (LAO) as part of the OCG examination?

    a. Make the exposure after full inhalation.
    b. Rotate large patients more than thin patients.
    c. Rotate thin patients more than large patients.
    d. Center the cassette to the left upper quadrant.

46. Which procedure should be performed for the right lateral decubitus position as part of the OCG examination?

    a. Place the patient on a radiolucent cushion.
    b. Center the cassette to the level of the iliac crests.
    c. Use a marker to indicate that the right side of the patient is the side up.
    d. Place the patient in the lateral recumbent position with the left side down.

47. What is an advantage of performing the right lateral decubitus position to demonstrate the gall bladder?

    a. It enables the gall bladder to be removed from the liver.
    b. It enables the stomach to provide a homogeneous background density.
    c. It enables the gall bladder to gravitate toward the dependent left side of the abdomen.
    d. It enables the gall bladder to gravitate toward the dependent right side of the abdomen.

48. Which two projections best visualize the stratification of gallstones?

    a. KUB and prone PA
    b. KUB and upright PA
    c. right lateral decubitus and prone PA
    d. right lateral decubitus and upright PA

49. Which position is generally not used as part of the OCG examination?

    a. PA
    b. LAO
    c. dorsal decubitus
    d. right lateral decubitus

50. Which projection/position of the gall bladder can be performed only with a horizontally directed central ray?

    a. PA
    b. LAO
    c. right lateral
    d. right lateral decubitus

If your school has access to Mosby's Radiographic Instructional Series on Anatomy, Positioning, and Procedures, review Unit 16 at this time; your instructor may request that you respond to the series' exercises on paper. This unit covers the following essential projections:

Abdomen
>   AP
>   PA, upright
>   AP, L lateral decubitus
>   Lateral, R or L
>   Lateral, R or L dorsal decubitus

Biliary tract and gall bladder
>   PA
>   PA oblique, LAO
>   Lateral, R only
>   AP, R lateral decubitus

Chapter 17
THE DIGESTIVE SYSTEM: THE ALIMENTARY TRACT

──────── Part 1

ANATOMY OF THE ALIMENTARY TRACT

Exercise 1

Instructions: This exercise pertains to the digestive system. Items require you to identify structures.

1. Identify each lettered structure in Figure 17-1.

A. _____

B. _____

C. _____

D. _____

E. _____

F. _____

G. _____

H. _____

I. _____

J. _____

K. _____

L. _____

M. _____

N. _____

O. _____

P. _____

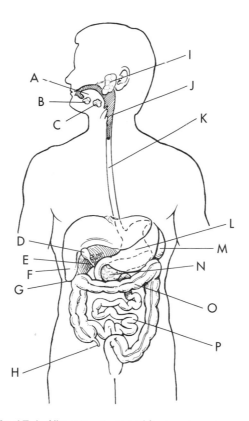

Fig. 17-1. Alimentary tract and its accessory organs.

2. Identify each lettered structure in Figure 17-2.

A. _____

B. _____

C. _____

D. _____

E. _____

F. _____

G. _____

H. _____

I. _____

J. _____

K. _____

L. _____

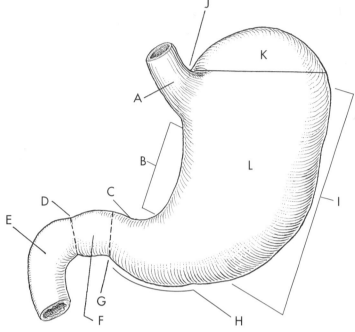

Fig. 17-2. Anterior surface of the stomach.

3. Identify each lettered structure in Figure 17-3.

A. _____

B. _____

C. _____

D. _____

E. _____

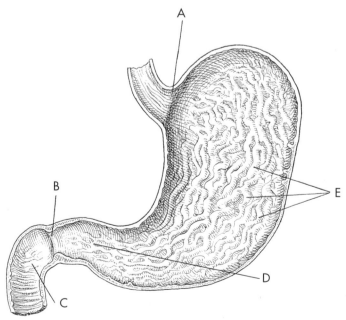

Fig. 17-3. Section of the stomach showing rugae.

4. Identify each lettered structure in Figure 17-4.

A. _____

B. _____

C. _____

D. _____

E. _____

F. _____

G. _____

H. _____

I. _____

J. _____

K. _____

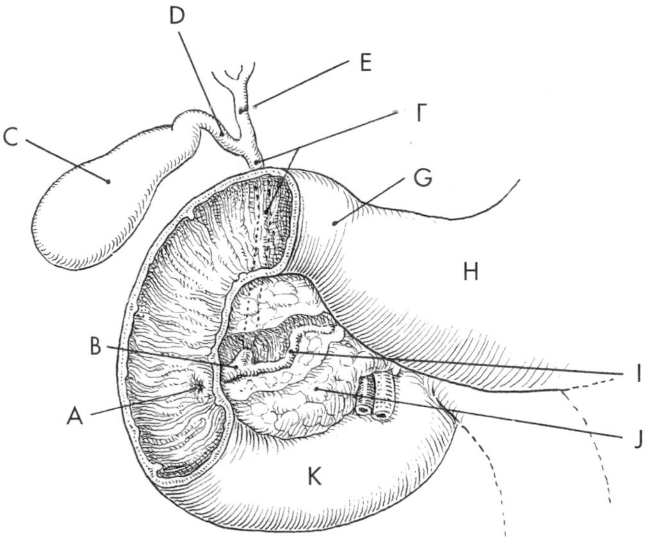

Fig. 17-4. Duodenal loop in relation to biliary and pancreatic ducts.

5. Identify each lettered structure in Figure 17-5.

A. _____

B. _____

C. _____

D. _____

E. _____

F. _____

G. _____

H. _____

I. _____

J. _____

K. _____

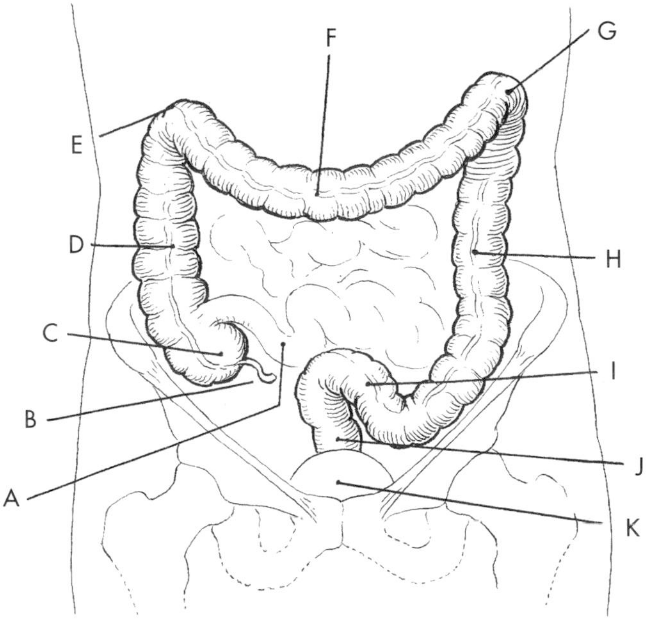

Fig. 17-5. Anterior aspect of the large bowel.

6. Identify each lettered structure in Figure 17-6.

A. _____

B. _____

C. _____

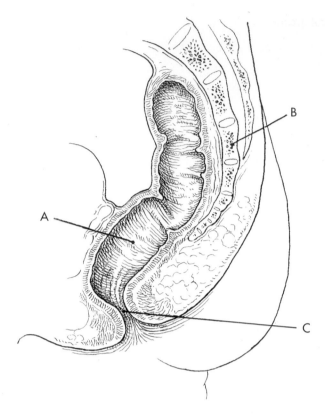

Fig. 17-6. Sagittal section showing anal canal and rectum.

Exercise 2

Instructions: Use the following clues to complete the crossword puzzle below. All answers refer to the alimentary tract.

ACROSS

1. Stores bile
5. Gastric folds
8. Attached to cecum
10. Terminates alimentary tract
11. Widest part of alimentary tract
15. Contraction waves
18. Proximal part of small bowel
19. Left colic flexure
22. Between cecum and hepatic flexure
23. Average body build
24. Precedes anal canal

DOWN

2. Digestive juice
3. Musculomembranous tube
4. Upper part of stomach
6. Lower than sthenic
7. Proximal part of large intestine
9. Precedes esophagus
12. Large body build
13. Middle part of small bowel
14. Very slender body build
16. Intestinal bend
17. Between splenic and sigmoid
20. Produces bile
21. Distal part of small bowel

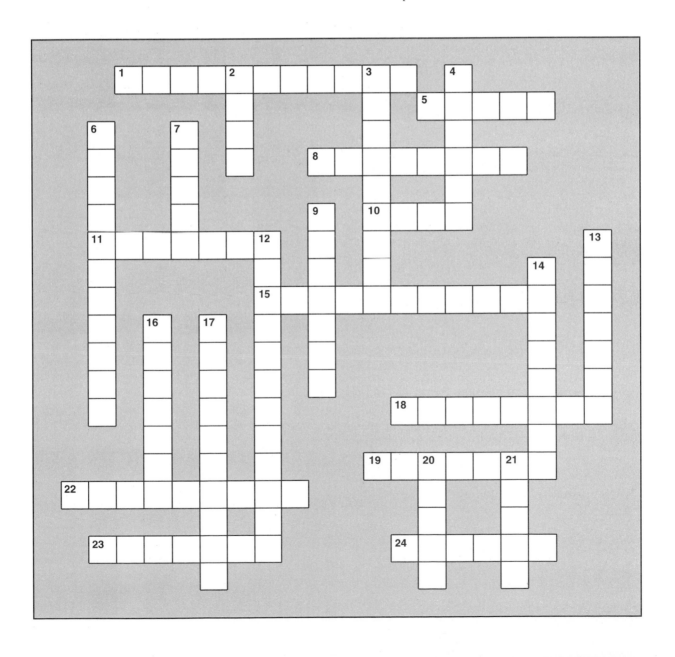

Exercise 3

Instructions: Match the structures or portions of organs found in the alimentary tract in Column A with the major organs to which they most closely relate in Column B.

Column A

____ 1. bulb

____ 2. body

____ 3. cecum

____ 4. ileum

____ 5. rugae

____ 6. rectum

____ 7. fundus

____ 8. jejunum

____ 9. pylorus

____ 10. sigmoid

____ 11. duodenum

____ 12. ascending

____ 13. descending

____ 14. transverse

____ 15. hepatic flexure

____ 16. ampulla of Vater

____ 17. lesser curvature

____ 18. greater curvature

____ 19. cardiac sphincter

____ 20. left colic flexure

Column B

a. stomach

b. small intestine

c. large intestine

Exercise 4

Instructions: This exercise pertains to the alimentary tract and its related organs. Items require you to fill in missing words or provide a short answer.

1. The musculomembranous passage that extends from the pharynx to the stomach is called the _____.

2. The expanded part of the distal end of the esophagus is the _____ _____.

3. The opening into the stomach through which food and liquids pass is the _____ _____.

4. The organ in which gastric digestion begins is the _____.

5. The gastric folds of the stomach are the _____.

6. What border of the stomach is the lesser curvature?

7. The lesser curvature extends from the esophagogastric junction to the _____.

8. The left and inferior borders of the stomach are the _____ _____.

9. Figure 17-7 shows four diagrams, each representing a different body habitus. Indicate below which of the following types each diagram represents: sthenic, asthenic, hyposthenic, or hypersthenic.

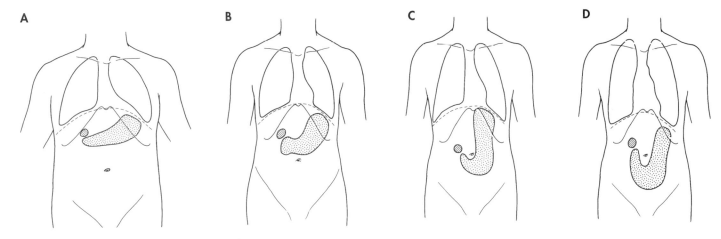

Fig. 17-7. The four types of body habitus.

a. Diagram A: _____

b. Diagram B: _____

c. Diagram C: _____

d. Diagram D: _____

10. Name the four parts of the stomach.

11. The part of the stomach that immediately surrounds the esophageal opening is the _____.

12. The most superior part of the stomach is the _____.

13. The most inferior part of the stomach is the _____ portion.

14. The opening between the stomach and the small intestine is the _____ _____.

15. Name the three parts of the small intestine.

16. The proximal part of the small intestine is the _____.

17. The first segment of the proximal part of the small intestine is radiographically significant; it is the _____

    _____.

18. The small intestine terminates at the _____ _____.

19. What part of the alimentary tract do the common bile ducts and the pancreatic ducts empty into?

20. The middle part of the small intestine is the _____.

21. The distal part of the small intestine is the _____.

22. What part of the small intestine is the shortest? the longest?

23. Which is longer, the small intestine or the large intestine?

24. The passage from the small intestine to the large intestine is the _____ _____.

25. The proximal part of the large intestine is the _____.

26. The appendix is attached to the large intestine at the _____.

27. Another name for the hepatic flexure is the _____ _____ _____.

28. The part of the colon that extends from the cecum to the right colic flexure is the _____ _____.

29. The part of the large intestine that extends between the two flexures is the _____ _____.

30. Another name for the splenic flexure is the _____ _____ _____.

31. What part of the colon extends inferiorly from the left colic flexure?

32. Between what two parts of the large intestine is the sigmoid colon found?

33. The sigmoid colon terminates in the _____.

34. What part of the large intestine extends between the rectum and the anus?

35. The external opening of the terminal end of the anal canal is the _____.

—————————— Part 2

POSITIONING OF THE ALIMENTARY TRACT

Exercise 1 Positioning for the Esophagus

Instructions: The esophagus can be radiographically examined after a contrast medium is introduced. This exercise pertains to procedures for obtaining the required radiographs of the esophagus. Items require you to fill in missing words, provide a short answer, or choose true or false. Explain any statement you believe is false.

1. True or False. Single-contrast and double-contrast studies can be used to demonstrate the esophagus.

2. True or False. A barium sulfate mixture is the contrast medium of choice for esophagrams.

3. True or False. The most important requirement for the contrast medium is that it be rated greater than 50% weight/volume.

4. What two contrast media are used for the double-contrast esophageal study?

5. List the projections that comprise the typical esophageal study.

6. Why is an LAO position not included in the typical esophageal study?

7. To demonstrate the entire esophagus, to what level of the patient should the cassette be centered?

8. What two obliques can be used to effectively demonstrate the entire esophagus?

9. For the PA (anterior) oblique position, the patient should be rotated approximately _____ to _____ degrees.

10. Why is the recumbent RAO position preferred over the upright position?

11. For the AP or PA projection, how is it determined that the selection of exposure factors was acceptable?

12. In relation to surrounding structures, where should the esophagus appear in the image with the patient in the RAO position?

13. In the radiograph of the contrast-filled esophagus with the patient positioned RAO, how does the esophagus appear, in relation to surrounding structures, when there was insufficient rotation of the patient?

14. In the radiograph of the lateral projection, what structures are used to determine whether the patient was rotated, and how should they appear?

15. The esophagus should be clearly seen from the lower neck to the _____ _____.

Exercise 2 The Gastrointestinal Series

Instructions: One of the more commonly performed studies employing contrast media is the gastrointestinal series. This exercise pertains to the GI study. Items require you to identify structures, fill in missing words, provide a short answer, or choose true or false. Explain any statement you believe is false.

Items 1 through 20 pertain to upper gastrointestinal examination procedures.

1. What two acronyms refer to the routine upper gastrointestinal series?

2. As part of patient preparation, why should the patient follow a soft, low-residue diet for two days?

3. How can the UGI study be affected if the patient smokes cigarettes shortly before the examination?

4. What type of radiopaque contrast medium is usually used in routine UGI studies?

5. List the two general GI examination procedures routinely used to examine the stomach.

6. What is the range of weight/volume concentration for the barium sulfate suspension usually used for single-contrast examinations?

7. What are the two types of contrast media used with the double-contrast procedure?

8. List two advantages of performing the double-contrast examination.

9. True or False. Both the single-contrast procedure and the double-contrast procedure should begin with the patient lateral recumbent.

10. True or False. The barium sulfate suspension used for the double-contrast examination should have higher weight/volume ratio than the barium sulfate suspension used for the single-contrast examination.

11. True or False. After the patient consumes the barium sulfate suspension for the double-contrast examination, all radiographs should be performed with the patient in the upright position.

12. Why should the patient undergoing the double-contrast examination turn from side to side or roll over a few times during the procedure?

13. What role does glucagon have during the double-contrast examination?

14. During the double-contrast examination, what instructions should be given, after the patient swallows the carbon dioxide crystals or tablets, to ensure a double-contrast effect?

15. What is a biphasic GI examination?

16. Which method of examination—the single-contrast or the double-contrast—is performed first as part of a biphasic examination?

17. List the two methods of performing hypotonic duodenography.

18. True or False. Hypotonic duodenography originally required the contrast medium to be directly introduced through a tube placed into the duodenum.

19. True or False. The tubeless hypotonic duodenography examination is performed after the duodenum has been temporarily paralyzed by a drug.

20. True or False. Hypotonic duodenography has largely been replaced by other imaging modalities, such as sonography and computed tomography.

Items 21 through 31 pertain to the PA projection.

21. True or False. Routine radiographs of the stomach and duodenum should be made with the patient in the upright position.

22. True or False. The PA projection with the patient prone demonstrates the contour of the barium-filled stomach and duodenal bulb.

23. True or False. The upright PA projection shows the size, shape, and relative position of the barium-filled stomach.

24. True or False. A compression band may be used across the abdomen to immobilize the patient and reduce involuntary movement of the viscera.

25. How should the prone position of the patient be adjusted to prevent the full weight of the abdomen from causing the stomach and duodenum to press against the vertebral column?

26. Describe the centering of a 10- X 12-inch (24- X 30-cm) cassette.

27. Describe the centering of a 14- X 17-inch (35- X 43-cm) cassette.

28. Describe how the centering of the film should be adjusted if the patient is repositioned from the prone to the upright position.

29. The greatest visceral movement between the prone and upright positions occurs in the _____ body habitus.

30. The central ray should be directed perpendicularly to enter the patient at the level of _____.

31. At the end of what phase of respiration should the exposure be made?

Items 32 through 37 pertain to the right PA oblique (RAO) projection.

32. Describe how the patient is adjusted from the prone position to the RAO position.

33. How many degrees should the patient be rotated from the prone position?

34. What type of body habitus requires the most rotation?

35. Where should the central ray enter the patient?

36. True or False. For the average patient, the RAO position produces the best image of the pyloric canal and the duodenal bulb filled with barium.

37. True or False. The RAO projection radiograph should be exposed after the patient suspends respiration after full inhalation.

Items 38 through 44 pertain to the left AP oblique (LPO) projection.

38. The LPO position is best performed if the patient is adjusted from the _____ position.

39. What side of the patient is elevated away from the table?

40. Most patients should be rotated _____ degrees.

41. Where should the central ray enter the patient?

42. True or False. The LPO position demonstrates the fundic portion of the stomach filled with barium.

43. True or False. The LPO position demonstrates the pyloric canal and duodenal bulb filled with barium.

44. Identify each lettered structure in Figure 17-8.

A. _____

B. _____

C. _____

D. _____

E. _____

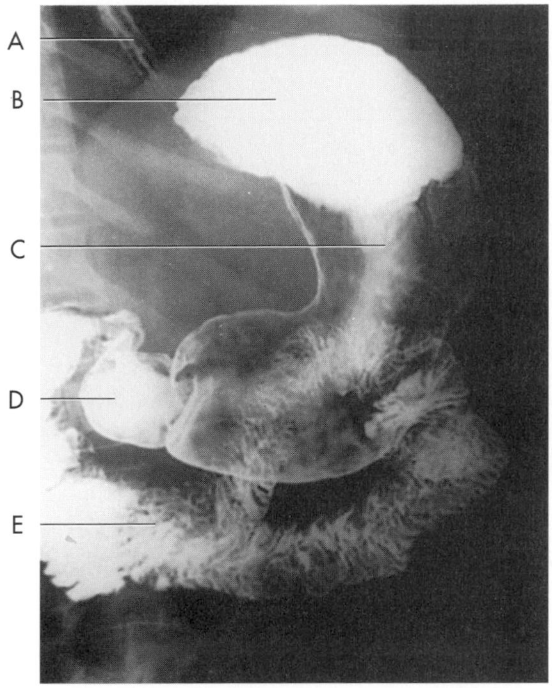

Fig. 17-8. LPO (left AP oblique) stomach and duodenum.

Items 45 through 50 pertain to the right lateral projection with the patient recumbent.

45. Indicate whether the following gastric structures are demonstrated mostly barium-filled or gas-filled:

a. Stomach fundus: _____

b. Duodenal bulb: _____

c. Duodenum: _____

46. What osteologic structures should be examined to determine whether the patient was rotated?

47. What two positioning landmarks that can be identified on the anterior surface of the body should be used to center the cassette?

48. The central ray should enter the patient at the level of the _____ vertebra.

49. If the recumbent patient is moved to the upright lateral position, to what level of the vertebrae should the central ray enter the patient?

50. Identify each lettered structure in Figure 17-9.

A. _____

B. _____

C. _____

D. _____

E. _____

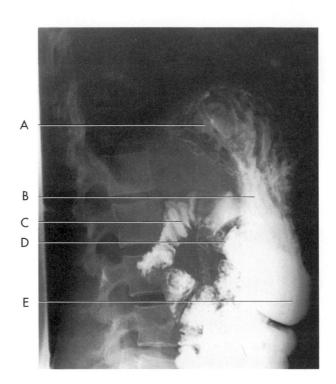

Fig. 17-9. LPO position.

Items 51 through 55 pertain to the AP projection.

51. The portion of the stomach that is demonstrated filled with barium is the _____.

52. Is the duodenum usually seen as barium-filled or gas-filled?

53. What gastric abnormality can be demonstrated by tilting the patient and table into the Trendelenburg position?

54. Describe the centering of the cassette for each of the following sizes:

a. 11 X 14 inches (30 X 35 cm):

b. 14 X 17 inches (35 X 43 cm):

55. Identify each lettered structure in Figure 17-10.

A. _____

B. _____

C. _____

D. _____

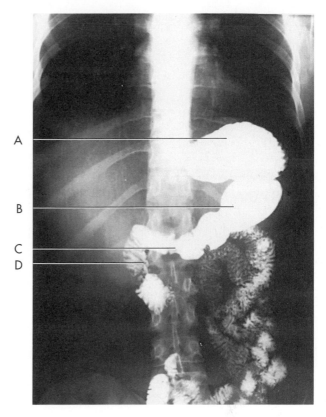

Fig. 17-10. AP stomach and duodenum.

Exercise 3 The Small Intestine Examination

Instructions: The small intestine can be radiographically examined by more than one method, often after the stomach is examined. This exercise pertains to the study of the small intestine, often referred to as the small bowel series. Items require you to provide a short answer.

1. List the three methods by which the barium sulfate mixture can be administered for a small bowel series.

2. What method of performing a small bowel series is most commonly used?

3. What method of performing a small bowel series often requires the administration of glucagon or Valium to relax the intestine and reduce patient discomfort during the initial filling of the small intestine?

4. Into what body position should the patient be placed when the small intestine is filled by the complete reflux method?

5. Define *enteroclysis*.

6. Into what part of the small intestine should the tube be inserted for the enteroclysis method of performing a small bowel series?

7. What patient preparation should be accomplished before the examination begins?

8. What method of performing a small bowel series should not use a cleansing enema as part of patient preparation?

9. Why is a time marker displayed on each radiograph taken during a small bowel series?

10. Into what body position should the patient be placed for timed radiographs?

11. Approximately how long after the patient swallows the barium sulfate mixture should the first radiograph be made?

12. Approximately how long after the first radiograph is taken should subsequent radiographs be exposed?

13. Why might the patient be given a cup of cold water to drink during the oral method of small bowel examination?

14. The visualization of what structure usually indicates that the entire small intestine has been adequately demonstrated?

15. List the seven evaluation criteria that indicate the small bowel series radiographs are properly performed.

Exercise 4 The Large Intestine Examination

Instructions: The large intestine is frequently examined radiographically after the introduction of a suitable contrast medium; this examination is called the barium enema (BE). This exercise pertains to the procedures and radiographs for the two methods of barium enemas. Items require you to identify structures, fill in missing words, provide a short answer, match columns, or choose true or false. Explain any statement you believe is false.

1. List the two basic methods of performing a barium enema.

2. What is the most common type of contrast medium used for BEs?

3. Why should a high-density barium product be the contrast medium of choice for the double-contrast study?

4. What two radiolucent contrast media can be used during the double-contrast study?

5. When might an orally administered, water-soluble, iodinated contrast medium be used in place of a barium sulfate mixture?

6. What is the general patient preparation for the BE?

7. What is considered the most important aspect of patient preparation for the BE?

8. What temperature should the barium be when it is desirable to administer warm barium solution?

9. How could the patient be affected if the barium solution is too warm?

10. What temperature should the barium be when it is desirable to administer cold barium solution?

11. What are the advantages of filling the large intestine with a cold barium solution?

12. List three instructions that can be given to the patient to help the patient better retain the barium during the examination.

13. What is the maximum distance that the enema tip should be inserted into the patient?

14. An IV stand used to hold the BE bag should be adjusted to place the bag approximately _____ to _____ inches above the level of the anus.

15. The last BE radiograph usually taken is called the _____ film.

16. The PA projection should be made with the patient in the _____ position.

17. For the AP or PA projection, the cassette should be centered to the patient at the level of the _____

    _____.

18. For the PA projection, the central ray should be directed _____ to the center of the film.

19. Identify each lettered structure in Figure 17-11.

A. _____ (flexure)

B. _____ (flexure)

C. _____

D. _____

E. _____

F. _____

G. _____

H. _____

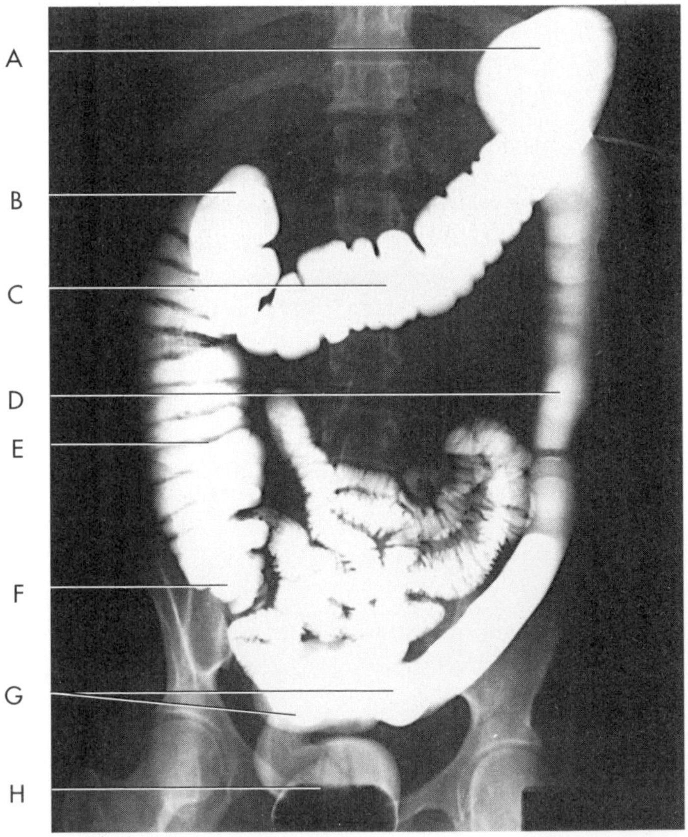

Fig. 17-11. PA colon.

20. The PA axial projection is used to demonstrate the _____ area of the large intestine.

21. How many degrees and in which direction should the central ray be directed for the PA axial projection?

22. To what level of the patient should the central ray be directed for the PA axial projection?

23. For the PA axial projection, what plane of the body should be centered to the midline of the table?

24. Identify each lettered structure in Figure 17-12.

A. _____ (flexure)

B. _____

C. _____

D. _____

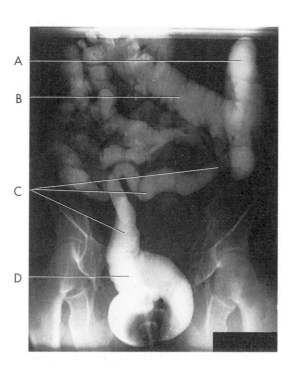

Fig. 17-12. PA axial large intestine.

25. True or False. Both colic flexures should be seen with the PA axial projection.

26. True or False. Both colic flexures should be seen in the RAO position radiograph.

27. True or False. The RAO position is performed primarily to demonstrate the right colic (hepatic) flexure.

28. True or False. For the RAO position, the central ray should be directed 35 to 45 degrees caudally.

29. True or False. For the RAO position, the patient should be rotated 35 to 45 degrees from the prone position.

30. Identify each lettered structure in Figure 17-13.

A. _____ (flexure)

B. _____ (flexure)

C. _____

D. _____

E. _____

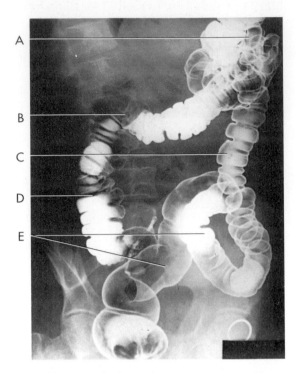

Fig. 17-13. RAO (right PA oblique) large intestine.

31. What two structures of the large intestine are primarily demonstrated with the left anterior oblique position?

32. To what level of the patient should the cassette be centered for the left PA oblique projection (LAO)?

33. Identify each lettered structure in Figure 17-14.

A. _____ (flexure)

B. _____ (flexure)

C. _____

D. _____

E. _____

F. _____

G. _____

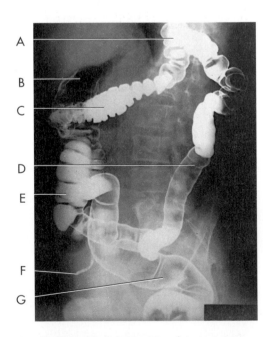

Fig. 17-14. LAO (left PA oblique) large intestine.

34. For the right or left lateral projection, to what level of the patient should a 10- X 12-inch (24- X 30-cm) cassette be centered?

35. In the image of the left lateral projection, how is it determined that the patient was not rotated?

36. The right or left lateral projection is performed to demonstrate the _____ and _____ portions of the large intestine.

37. For a lateral projection to demonstrate the rectum and sigmoid portions, what plane of the body should be centered to the midline of the table?

38. Identify each lettered structure in Figure 17-15.

A. _____

B. _____

C. _____

D. _____

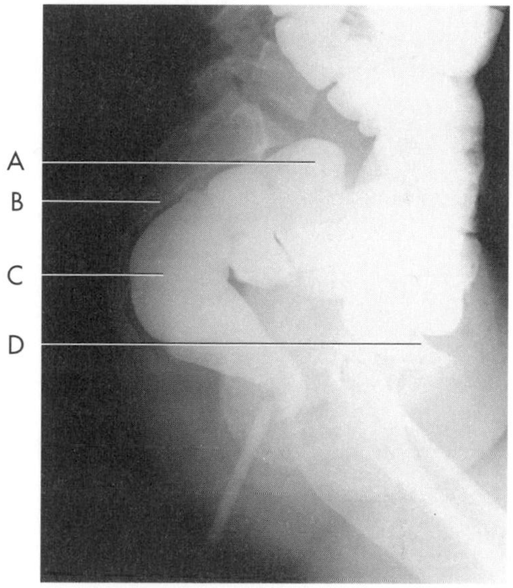

Fig. 17-15. Lateral position.

39. The AP axial projection produces an image similar to the _____ _____ projection.

40. For the AP axial projection, the central ray should be directed _____ at an angle of _____ to _____ degrees.

41. For the AP axial projection, where on the patient's anterior surface should the central ray enter when a 14- X 17-inch (35- X 43-cm) film is used?

42. To produce a coned-down image of the AP axial projection on a 10- X 12-inch (24- X 30-cm) film, where on the patient should the central ray enter?

43. Identify each lettered structure in Figure 17-16.

A. _____

B. _____

C. _____

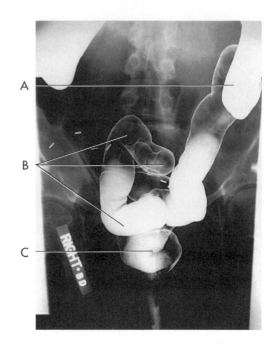

Fig. 17-16. AP axial large intestine.

44. The LPO position produces an image similar to the _____ position.

45. For the LPO position, the patient should be rotated _____ to _____ degrees.

46. For the LPO position, what side of the patient should be elevated away from the x-ray table?

47. What flexure should be well demonstrated with the LPO position?

48. Identify each lettered structure in Figure 17-17.

A. _____ (flexure)

B. _____ (flexure)

C. _____

D. _____

E. _____

F. _____

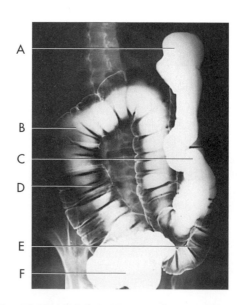

Fig. 17-17. LPO (left AP oblique) large intestine.

49. What other oblique position produces an image similar to the LAO position?

50. What flexure should be well demonstrated with the RPO position?

51. How many degrees should the patient be rotated from the supine position for the RPO position?

52. Identify each lettered structure in Figure 17-18.

A. _____

B. _____

C. _____

D. _____

E. _____

F. _____

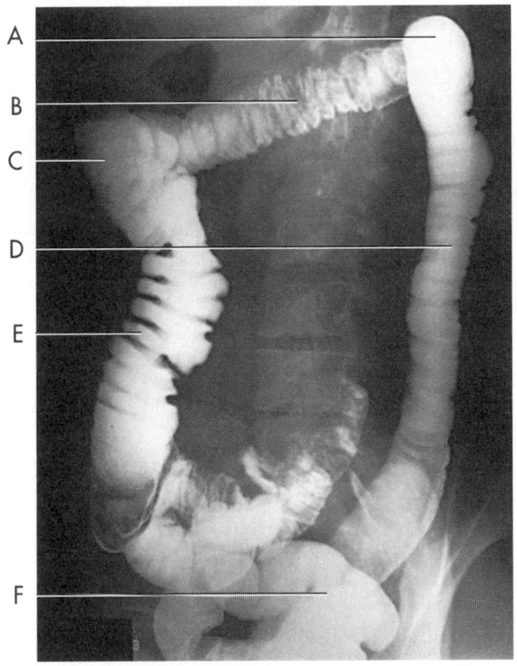

Fig. 17-18. RPO (right AP oblique) large intestine.

53. What BE radiograph requires the patient positioned right lateral recumbent and a horizontal central ray directed to the midline of the patient at the level of the iliac crests?

54. For a lateral decubitus position, what should be accomplished to ensure that the dependent side of the patient is demonstrated?

55. Name the lateral decubitus position that best demonstrates each of the following intestinal structures:

a. Left colic (splenic) flexure: _____

b. Right colic (hepatic) flexure: _____

56. Figures 17-19 and 17-20 are lateral decubitus projection radiographs. Examine the images and answer the questions that follow.

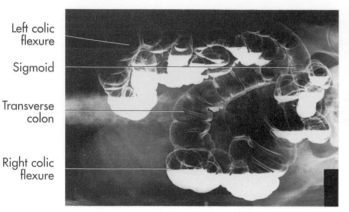

Left colic
flexure

Sigmoid

Transverse
colon

Right colic
flexure

Fig. 17-19. Lateral decubitus position.

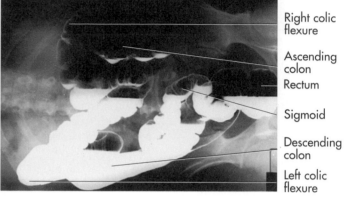

Right colic
flexure

Ascending
colon

Rectum

Sigmoid

Descending
colon

Left colic
flexure

Fig. 17-20. Lateral decubitus position, PA large intestine.

a. Which image shows the left lateral decubitus position?

b. Which image shows the right lateral decubitus position?

c. Which image best demonstrates the left colic (splenic) flexure?

d. Which image best demonstrates the right colic (hepatic) flexure?

e. Which image requires the patient to be placed in the left lateral recumbent position?

f. Which image requires the patient to be placed in the right lateral recumbent position?

57. How much of the colon should be demonstrated in the image of a lateral decubitus position?

58. For upright frontal, oblique, and lateral projections, how is the centering of the film adjusted from that used for the recumbent positions? Why is the compensation necessary?

59. Examine Figure 17-21 and answer the questions that follow.

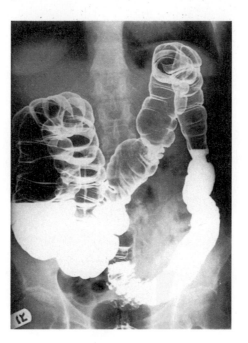

Fig. 17-21. AP position.

a. What body position was used to make this radiograph?

b. What image characteristics led you to that conclusion?

60. Figures 17-22 through 17-29 represent different projections/positions used to obtain BE radiographs. Examine the images, then match the figures in Column A with the positions in Column B.

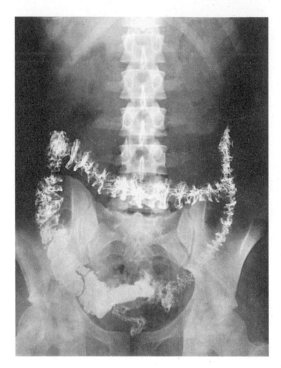

Fig. 17-22. BE radiograph.

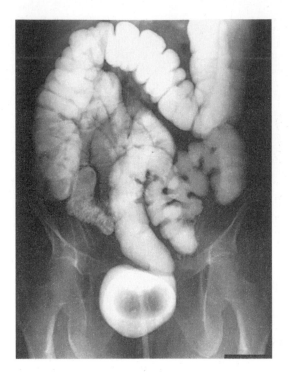

Fig. 17-23. BE radiograph.

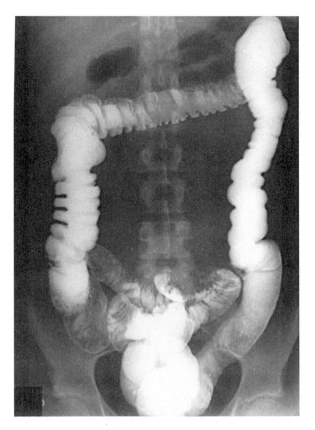

Fig. 17-24. BE radiograph.

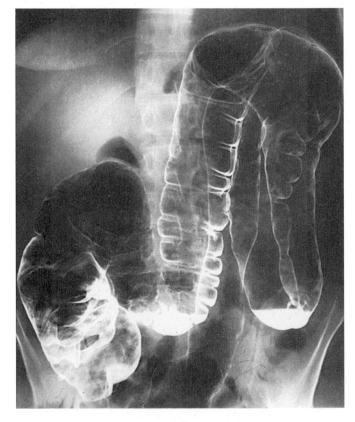

Fig. 17-25. BE radiograph.

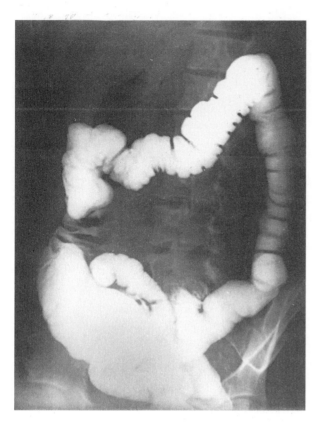

Fig. 17-26. BE radiograph.

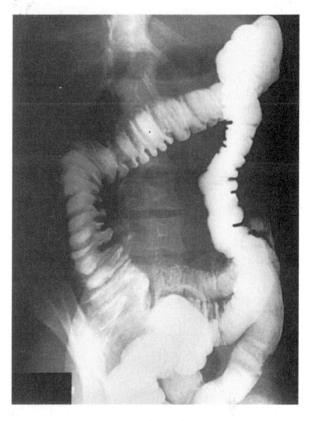

Fig. 17-27. BE radiograph.

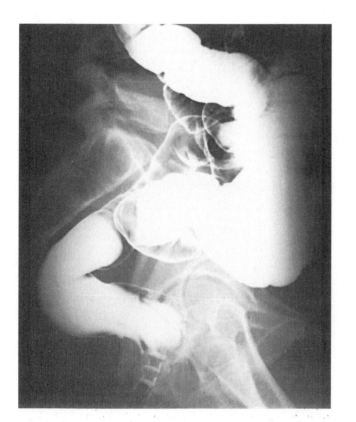

Fig. 17-28. BE radiograph.

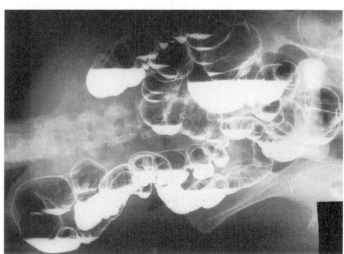

Fig. 17-29. BE radiograph.

Column A

____ 1. Figure 17-22

____ 2. Figure 17-23

____ 3. Figure 17-24

____ 4. Figure 17-25

____ 5. Figure 17-26

____ 6. Figure 17-27

____ 7. Figure 17-28

____ 8. Figure 17-29

Column B

a. LAO

b. LPO

c. AP axial

d. PA upright

e. AP recumbent

f. left lateral

g. post-evacuation

h. lateral decubitus

Self-Test: Anatomy and Positioning of the Alimentary Tract

Instructions: Answer the following questions by selecting the best choice.

1. Which body habitus type positions the stomach almost horizontal and high in the abdomen?

   a. sthenic
   b. asthenic
   c. hyposthenic
   d. hypersthenic

2. Which curvature is located on the right (medial) border of the stomach?

   a. lesser
   b. greater
   c. superior
   d. inferior

3. What is the most superior part of the stomach?

   a. head
   b. body
   c. fundus
   d. pylorus

4. What is the most inferior part of the stomach?

   a. body
   b. cardia
   c. fundus
   d. pylorus

5. The distal esophagus empties its contents into the:

   a. duodenum.
   b. duodenal bulb.
   c. pyloric canal.
   d. cardiac antrum.

6. Which opening is between the stomach and the small intestine?

   a. cardiac orifice
   b. pyloric orifice
   c. ampulla of Vater
   d. ileocecal orifice

7. Which opening is at the distal end of the small intestine?

   a. anus
   b. cardiac orifice
   c. pyloric orifice
   d. ileocecal orifice

8. Which structure is the proximal part of the small intestine?

   a. ileum
   b. jejunum
   c. pylorus
   d. duodenum

9. Which structure is the distal part of the small intestine?

   a. cecum
   b. ileum
   c. jejunum
   d. duodenum

10. In which abdominal region does the large intestine originate?

    a. left iliac
    b. right iliac
    c. left lumbar
    d. right lumbar

11. Which structure is the proximal part of the large intestine?

    a. cecum
    b. ileum
    c. rectum
    d. sigmoid

12. Which part of the large intestine is located between the ascending and descending portions of the colon?

    a. cecum
    b. rectum
    c. sigmoid
    d. transverse colon

13. Which flexure is also known as the right colic flexure?

    a. splenic
    b. hepatic
    c. angular notch
    d. duodenojejunal

14. Where in the large intestine is the left colic flexure located?

    a. between the cecum and the ascending colon
    b. between the ascending and transverse colons
    c. between the transverse and descending colons
    d. between the descending colon and the sigmoid

15. Which structure is the pouch-like part of the large intestine situated below the junction of the ileum and the colon?

    a. cecum
    b. rectum
    c. sigmoid
    d. appendix

16. Where in the large intestine is the sigmoid located?

    a. between the cecum and the transverse colon
    b. between the ascending and transverse colons
    c. between the transverse and descending colons
    d. between the descending colon and the rectum

17. Approximately how long does it take a barium meal to reach the ileocecal valve?

    a. 30 minutes to 1 hour
    b. 2 to 3 hours
    c. 4 to 5 hours
    d. 24 hours

18. How long does it generally take a barium meal to reach the rectum?

    a. 2 to 3 hours
    b. 4 to 5 hours
    c. 6 to 8 hours
    d. 24 hours

19. Which two imaging modalities are most commonly employed to examine the alimentary tract after the introduction of a barium product?

    a. fluoroscopy and sonography
    b. fluoroscopy and radiography
    c. computed tomography and sonography
    d. computed tomography and radiography

20. Which type of contrast medium is most commonly used for examining the upper gastrointestinal tract?

    a. an oily-viscous compound
    b. a barium sulfate suspension
    c. a nonionic injectable compound
    d. a water-soluble, iodinated solution

21. To best demonstrate the swallowing function, in which position should the patient be placed for beginning the fluoroscopic phase of the single-contrast examination of the esophagus?

    a. upright
    b. left lateral decubitus
    c. recumbent LAO
    d. recumbent RPO

22. Which two recumbent oblique positions can be used to best demonstrate an unobstructed image of a barium-filled esophagus between the vertebrae and the heart?

    a. LAO and LPO
    b. LAO and RPO
    c. RAO and LPO
    d. RAO and RPO

23. What is a major advantage of the double-contrast UGI examination over the single-contrast UGI examination?

    a. There is reduced radiation exposure to the patient.
    b. The patient can better tolerate the procedure.
    c. Small lesions on the mucosal lining are better demonstrated.
    d. The examination can be performed with the patient upright instead of recumbent.

24. Which description refers to the biphasic gastrointestinal examination?

    a. a single-contrast study of the entire alimentary tract
    b. a single-contrast study of the upper gastrointestinal tract
    c. a double-contrast study of the upper gastrointestinal tract
    d. a combination single- and double-contrast study of the upper gastrointestinal tract

25. Which body habitus produces the greatest visceral movement when a patient is moved from the prone to the upright position?

    a. sthenic
    b. asthenic
    c. hyposthenic
    d. hypersthenic

26. For the double-contrast UGI examination, which position produces the best image of a gas-filled duodenal bulb and pyloric canal?

    a. LPO with the patient upright
    b. RAO with the patient upright
    c. LPO with the patient recumbent
    d. RAO with the patient recumbent

27. For the single-contrast UGI examination, which projection/position with the patient recumbent produces the best image of a barium-filled duodenal bulb and pyloric canal?

    a. AP
    b. left lateral
    c. LPO (left AP oblique)
    d. RAO (right PA oblique)

28. Which projection/position with the patient recumbent best stimulates gastric peristalsis to better demonstrate the pyloric canal and duodenal bulb during the UGI examination?

    a. AP
    b. left lateral
    c. LPO (left AP oblique)
    d. RAO (right PA oblique)

29. Which breathing procedure should be performed by the patient when UGI radiographs are exposed?

    a. suspended inhalation
    b. suspended exhalation
    c. slow, deep breathing
    d. quick panting breaths

30. For the double-contrast UGI examination, which projection with the patient recumbent produces the best image of a gas-filled fundus?

    a. LPO
    b. RAO
    c. left lateral
    d. left lateral decubitus

31. For the UGI examination, which projection with the patient recumbent best demonstrates the right retrogastric space?

    a. right lateral
    b. right lateral decubitus
    c. LPO
    d. RAO

32. For the AP projection with the patient supine as part of the UGI examination, which procedure should be performed to best demonstrate a diaphragmatic herniation (hiatal hernia)?

    a. Angle the central ray 30 to 35 degrees caudally.
    b. Tilt the table and patient into full Trendelenburg position.
    c. Have the patient suspend respiration after full inhalation.
    d. Place radiolucent cushions under the thorax to elevate the shoulders.

33. To which level of the patient should the central ray be directed for the RAO position as part of the UGI examination?

    a. T10
    b. T12
    c. L2
    d. L4

34. Which examination of the alimentary tract requires a series of radiographs taken at specific time intervals after the ingestion of the contrast medium?

    a. barium enema
    b. esophagography
    c. small bowel series
    d. upper gastrointestinal series

35. For a small bowel series when the patient has hypomotility of the small intestine, which procedure should be performed to accelerate peristalsis?

    a. Roll the patient 360 degrees.
    b. Have the patient drink a glass of ice water.
    c. Have the patient perform the Valsalva maneuver.
    d. Tilt the table and patient into full Trendelenburg position.

36. The visualization of which structure usually indicates the completion of a small bowel series?

    a. cecum
    b. ileum
    c. jejunum
    d. duodenum

37. Which procedure should be accomplished during a barium enema to relax the large intestine and enable better retention of the barium sulfate suspension?

    a. Have the patient perform the Valsalva maneuver.
    b. Administer warm (95° F) barium sulfate suspension.
    c. Administer cold (41° F) barium sulfate suspension.
    d. Raise the barium bag to 24 inches above the rectum.

38. Which procedure should be performed when the enema tip is inserted during a barium enema?

    a. Lubricate the tip with petroleum jelly.
    b. Ensure that the tip is inserted 2 to 4 inches (5 to 10 cm).
    c. Place the patient in the Trendelenburg position.
    d. Inflate the air-filled retention tip prior to insertion.

39. Before the enema tip is inserted during a barium enema, why should a small amount of barium sulfate mixture be allowed to run into a waste basket?

    a. to lubricate the enema tip
    b. to remove air from the tube
    c. to determine if the mixture is too warm or too cold
    d. to ensure that the consistency of the mixture is adequate

40. For the PA projection during a barium enema, what is the advantage of placing the x-ray table and patient in a slight Trendelenburg position?

    a. to demonstrate the ileocecal valve
    b. to enable more air to be injected into the colon
    c. to help separate overlapping loops of distal bowel
    d. to cause the transverse colon to move higher in the abdomen

41. Which structures of the large intestine are of primary interest with the AP axial or PA axial projections during a barium enema?

    a. sigmoid and rectum
    b. cecum and ileocecal valve
    c. left and right colic flexures
    d. ascending and descending colons

42. How many degrees and in which direction should the central ray be directed for the PA axial projection during a barium enema?

    a. 20 to 25 degrees caudad
    b. 20 to 25 degrees cephalad
    c. 30 to 40 degrees caudad
    d. 30 to 40 degrees cephalad

43. Which structure of the large intestine is of primary interest for the RAO position during a barium enema examination?

    a. anal canal
    b. descending colon
    c. left colic (splenic) flexure
    d. right colic (hepatic) flexure

44. Which two oblique positions can be performed to best demonstrate the left colic (splenic) flexure during a barium enema?

    a. LAO and LPO
    b. LAO and RPO
    c. RAO and LPO
    d. RAO and RPO

45. Which structure of the large intestine is best demonstrated if, from a supine position, the patient is rotated 45 degrees to move the left side of the abdomen away from the x-ray table during a barium enema?

    a. cecum
    b. ileum
    c. left colic (splenic) flexure
    d. right colic (hepatic) flexure

46. For the right lateral decubitus position as part of a barium enema, what should be done to ensure that the ascending colon is demonstrated in the image?

    a. Center the film to the iliac crests.
    b. Elevate the patient on a radiolucent support.
    c. Make the exposure after the patient suspends respiration.
    d. Tilt the table and patient into full Trendelenburg position.

47. What is the proper sequence for filling the large intestine with barium when performing a barium enema?

    a. rectum, sigmoid, ascending colon, transverse colon, and descending colon
    b. rectum, sigmoid, descending colon, transverse colon, and ascending colon
    c. sigmoid, rectum, ascending colon, transverse colon, and descending colon
    d. sigmoid, rectum, descending colon, transverse colon, and ascending colon

48. Which BE position requires a 10- x 12-inch (24- x 30-cm) cassette to be centered lengthwise approximately 2 to 3 inches (5 to 7.5 cm) above the level of the symphysis pubis in the median coronal plane?

    a. AP
    b. lateral
    c. LPO (left AP oblique)
    d. left lateral decubitus

49. Which BE follow-up projection/position usually does not require that both flexures be included in the image?

    a. AP
    b. lateral
    c. lateral decubitus
    d. RAO (right PA oblique)

50. For the PA projection as part of the UGI examination, why should the lower lung fields be included on a 14- x 17-inch (35- x 43-cm) film?

    a. to demonstrate pneumothorax
    b. to demonstrate a possible hiatal hernia
    c. to demonstrate fluid levels in the thorax
    d. to demonstrate the gas bubble in the fundus of the stomach

If your school has access to Mosby's Radiographic Instructional Series on Anatomy, Positioning, and Procedures, review Unit 17 at this time; your instructor may request that you respond to the series' exercises on paper. This unit covers the following essential projections:

Esophagus
    AP or PA
    PA oblique, RAO or LPO
    Lateral, R or L

Stomach and duodenum
    PA
    PA oblique, RAO
    AP oblique, LPO
    Lateral, R only
    AP

Small intestine
    PA or AP

Large intestine
    PA
    PA axial
    PA oblique, RAO
    PA oblique, LAO
    Lateral, R or L
    AP
    AP axial
    AP oblique, LPO
    AP oblique, RPO
    AP or PA, R lateral decubitus
    PA or AP, L lateral decubitus
    AP, PA, oblique or lateral: Upright

Chapter 18
THE URINARY SYSTEM

Part 1

ANATOMY OF THE URINARY SYSTEM

Exercise 1

Instructions: This exercise pertains to urinary structures. Items require you to identify structures.

1. Identify each lettered structure in Figure 18-1.

A. _____

B. _____

C. _____

D. _____

E. _____

F. _____

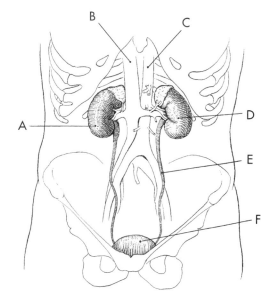

Fig. 18-1. Anterior aspect of urinary system in relation to surrounding structures.

2. Identify each lettered structure in Figure 18-2.

A. _____

B. _____

C. _____

D. _____

E. _____

F. _____

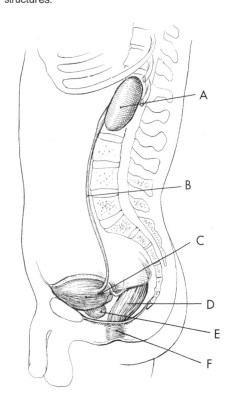

Fig. 18-2. Lateral aspect of the male urinary system in relation to surrounding structures.

3. Identify each lettered part of a kidney in Figure 18-3.

A. _____

B. _____

C. _____

D. _____

E. _____

F. _____

G. _____

H. _____

I. _____

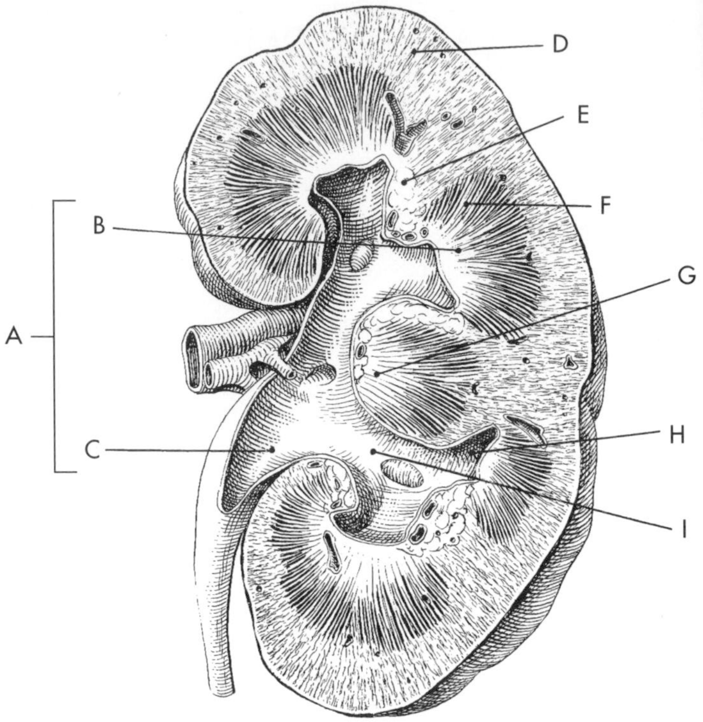

Fig. 18-3. Coronal section of a kidney.

4. Identify each lettered structure in Figure 18-4.

A. _____

B. _____

C. _____

D. _____

E. _____

F. _____

G. _____

H. _____

I. _____

J. _____

K. _____

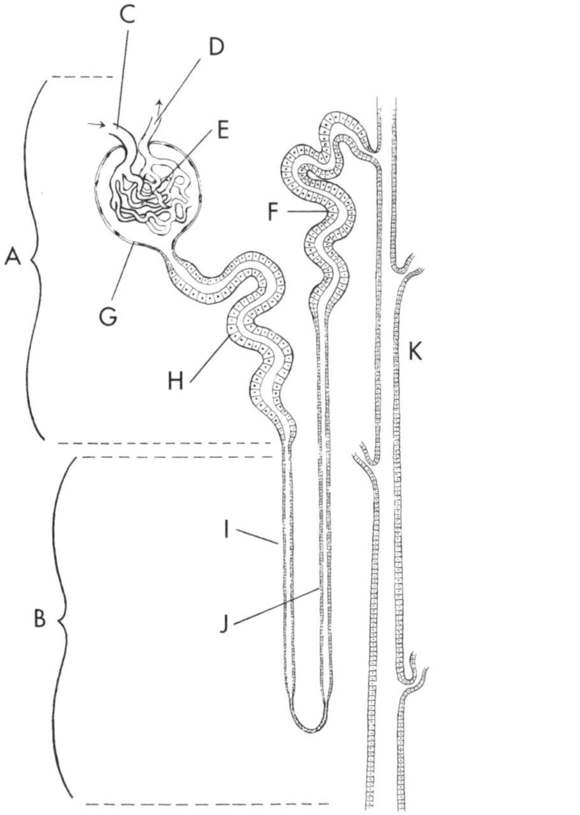

Fig. 18-4. Diagram of a nephron (renal corpuscle) and uriniferous tubule.

5. Identify each lettered structure in Figure 18-5.

A. _____

B. _____

C. _____

D. _____

E. _____

F. _____

G. _____

H. _____

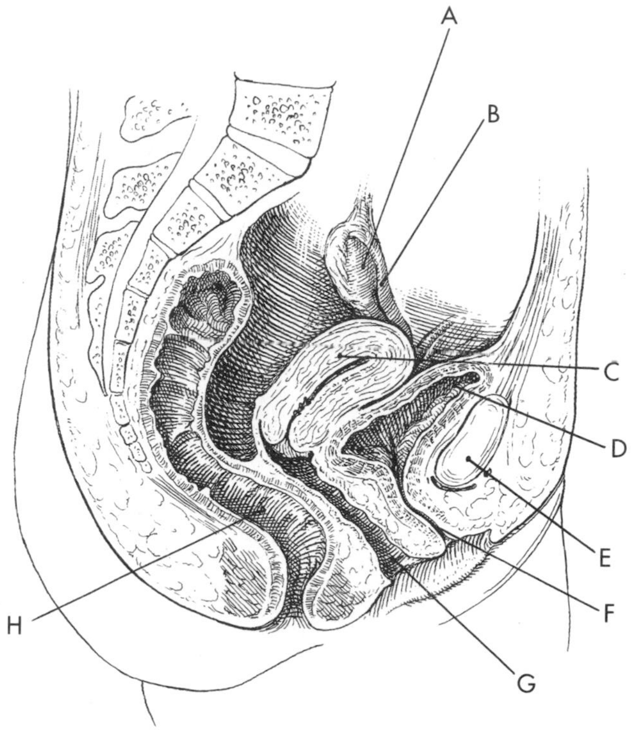

Fig. 18-5. Median sagittal section through the female pelvis.

6. Identify each lettered structure in Figure 18-6.

A. _____

B. _____

C. _____

D. _____

E. _____

F. _____

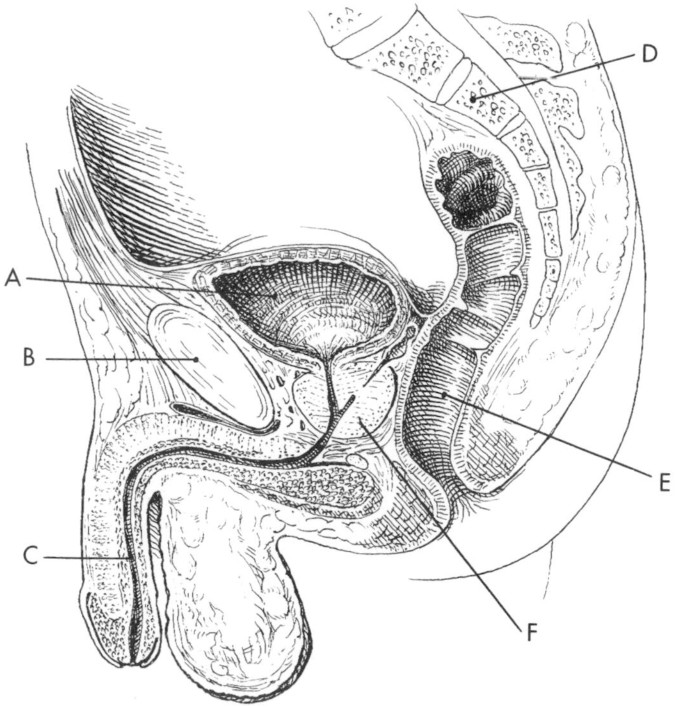

Fig. 18-6. Median sagittal section through the male pelvis.

Exercise 2

Instructions: Use the following clues to complete the crossword puzzle below. All answers refer to the urinary system.

ACROSS

3. Outer renal tissue
4. This arteriole leaves the capsule
6. Filtrate derivative
7. Another term for suprarenal
8. Urine vessel from glomerular capsule
10. Cup-shaped urine receivers
12. Cone-shaped renal segments
15. Cluster of blood vessels
16. Urinary reservoir
17. Functional renal unit
18. Musculomembranous excretory duct
19. Medial opening of a kidney

DOWN

1. This arteriole enters the capsule
2. Inner renal tissue
3. Membranous cup; Bowman's _____
5. Central renal cavity
6. External excretory tube
9. Male gland
11. This gland is found on a kidney
13. Glomerular fluid
14. Primary organ of urinary system

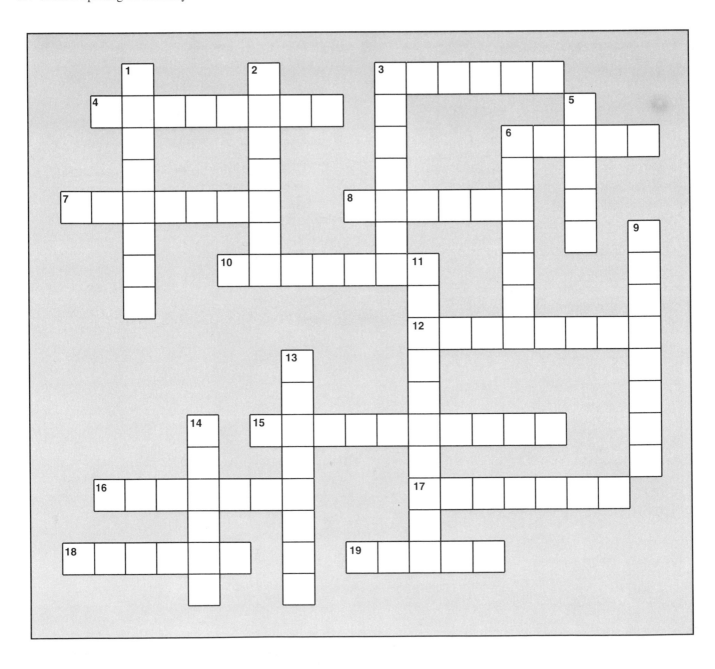

Exercise 3

Instructions: This exercise pertains to the anatomy of the urinary system. Items require you to fill in missing words or provide a short answer.

1. The kidneys and ureters belong to the _____ system.

2. What is the basic function of the kidneys?

3. What is the name of the gland that sits on the superior pole of each kidney?

4. Blood vessels, nerves, and the ureter enter a kidney through the opening known as the _____.

5. On what border of the kidney is the hilum found?

6. In the average (sthenic) person, the superior pole of the kidney is located at the _____ vertebral level.

7. The microscopic functional unit of the kidney is called the _____.

8. In what layer of renal tissue are nephron units found?

9. What is the name of the proximal portion of a nephron that consists of a double-walled membranous cup?

10. A cluster of blood capillaries that lie surrounded by a Bowman's capsule is called a _____.

11. A glomerulus branches off the _____ artery.

12. The blood vessel entering a glomerular capsule is the _____ arteriole, and the blood vessel leaving a glomerular capsule is the _____ arteriole.

13. The fluid that passes from the glomerulus to the glomerular capsule is called _____ _____ .

14. Urine from collecting ducts drains into minor _____.

15. Minor calyces drain urine into major _____.

16. Major calyces unite to form the expanded, funnel-shaped renal _____.

17. The long tubes that transport urine from the kidneys are called _____.

18. Ureters transport urine from kidneys to the _____ _____.

19. What is the name of the musculomembranous tube that conveys urine from the urinary bladder to outside the body?

20. The gland that surrounds the proximal part of the male urethra is called the _____.

Part 2

POSITIONING OF THE URINARY SYSTEM

Exercise 1 Excretory Urography

Instructions: Radiography of the urinary system comprises numerous specialized procedures. The most common radiographic examination of the urinary system is the excretory urogram. This exercise pertains to excretory urography. Items require you to identify structures, fill in missing words, or provide a short answer.

1. The radiographic investigation of the renal drainage system is accomplished by various procedures classified under the

   general term of _____.

2. List two other terms that refer to the excretory urogram examination.

3. What is the typical type of contrast medium currently used in excretory urography?

4. List mild and severe reactions that could occur after iodinated contrast medium has been intravenously injected into a patient.

   a. Mild reactions:

   b. Severe reactions:

5. How soon after the injection of a contrast medium are symptoms of a reaction likely to occur?

6. List four typical procedures the patient might experience in the ideal situation when preparing for the IVU examination.

7. What is the purpose of giving a child 12 ounces of carbonated beverage just prior to the start of IVU?

8. Why should an immobilization band not be applied across the patient's upper abdomen during IVU in an effort to control motion?

9. What is the purpose of applying compression over the distal ends of the ureters?

10. Where on the abdomen should compression pads be located when it is desirable to compress the ureters?

11. When ureteral compression is employed, why should the pressure be slowly released when the compression device is no longer needed?

12. Why is ureteral compression currently not often used in excretory urography?

13. Most excretory urograms should be exposed when the patient has suspended respiration after _____.

14. Prior to the injection of the contrast medium, why might an upright AP projection be made of the abdomen?

15. What identification data should be included on every post-injection radiograph?

16. Why should the patient be asked to empty the bladder just before IVU is to begin?

17. Why is it desirable to have the patient remove his or her underwear?

18. List five reasons that the AP projection with the patient recumbent is performed as the scout radiograph.

19. Why is it desirable to include the area below the symphysis pubis for older male patients?

20. When the recumbent patient is positioned for the AP projection, why should a support be placed under the knees?

21. What can be done to enhance the filling of renal structures with the contrast medium when the patient is supine?

22. What is the purpose of obtaining a radiograph 30 seconds after a bolus injection of the contrast medium?

23. How long after the completion of the contrast medium injection before the contrast agent usually begins to appear in the renal pelvis?

24. After injection of the contrast medium, the greatest concentration usually appears within the kidneys in _____ to _____ minutes.

25. What adjustment in the patient's position can be made to better demonstrate the distal ends of the ureters?

26. What procedure should be followed if the bladder is not seen in the AP projection to demonstrate the entire urinary system?

27. Approximately how many degrees should the patient be rotated from the supine position for an oblique position to demonstrate renal and urinary structures?

28. What positioning error most likely would cause a ureter to be seen superimposed with vertebrae in the LPO (left AP oblique) position?

29. A post-voiding radiograph is usually the last radiograph taken to demonstrate the _____.

30. Identify each lettered structure in Figure 18-7.

A. _____

B. _____

C. _____

D. _____

E. _____

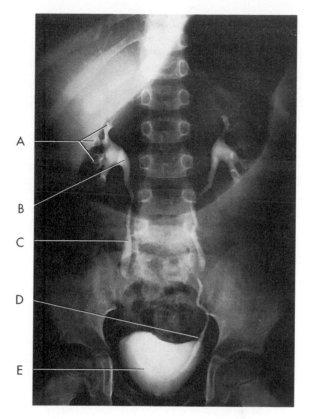

Fig. 18-7. AP projection of the urinary system.

Exercise 2 Retrograde Urography

Instructions: Retrograde urography is a radiographic procedure that demonstrates certain urinary structures. This exercise pertains to retrograde urography. Items require you to fill in missing words, provide a short answer, or choose true or false. Explain any statement you believe is false.

1. True or False. Retrograde urography differs from excretory urography in that the contrast medium is injected directly into the kidney by means of a percutaneous injection through the skin.

2. True or False. Retrograde urography is performed on a regular x-ray table.

3. At the beginning of the retrograde urographic examination, the patient is placed in the modified _____ position.

4. What size film is used to make the urograms?

5. Who should inject the contrast medium?

6. Describe how a kidney function test can be performed during retrograde urography.

7. List the three AP projection radiographs that usually comprise a retrograde urographic examination.

8. Why might the head of the x-ray table be lowered 10 to 15 degrees during the retrograde pyelography procedure?

9. What retrograde urographic radiograph can sometimes require the head of the table to be elevated 35 to 40 degrees?

10. After necessary AP projections are made, what oblique projections often are requested?

Exercise 3 Retrograde Cystography

Instructions: Projections obtained during retrograde cystography often include an AP, both AP obliques (RPO and LPO), and a lateral. This exercise pertains to those projections. Items require you to fill in missing words or provide a short answer.

1. Describe how the contrast medium is introduced into the patient for retrograde cystography.

2. What size film should be used to demonstrate the bladder, and how should it be placed in the cassette holder?

3. To what level of the patient should the cassette be centered for the AP projection?

4. Why should the patient extend the lower limbs for the AP projection?

5. List the three ways the central ray can be directed for the AP projection.

6. What positioning factor determines how the central ray should be directed for the AP projection?

7. How should the central ray be directed for the AP projection of the bladder as part of a voiding cystogram?

8. How far above the upper border of the symphysis pubis should the central ray enter the patient?

9. The exposure should be made after _____.

10. What structures are sometimes better demonstrated with the AP projection with the head of the table lowered 15 to 20 degrees and the central ray directed vertically?

11. State how the pubic bones should be demonstrated in the AP projection image.

12. How many degrees should the patient be rotated for the AP oblique projections?

13. List the two ways the central ray can be directed for the AP oblique projections.

14. How should the patient's uppermost thigh be positioned to prevent it superimposing the bladder in an AP oblique projection?

15. The following questions pertain to the lateral projection:

   a. The patient should be placed in the _____ _____ position.

   b. A cassette should be centered to the patient at a level 2 to 3 inches (5 to 7.5 cm) above the _____

   _____.

   c. The central ray should be directed _____.

Exercise 4   Male Cystourethrography

Instructions: This exercise pertains to male cystourethrography. Items require you to provide a short answer or choose true or false. Explain any statement you believe is false.

1. Define *cystourethrography*.

2. Describe how the contrast medium is introduced into the urinary structures of interest.

3. After the contrast medium is introduced into the patient, in what position is the patient placed to demonstrate urinary structures?

4. How many degrees should the patient be rotated for the desired oblique projection?

5. To what level of the patient should the cassette be centered?

6. To ensure adequate coverage, should the cassette be placed lengthwise or crosswise?

7. True or False. In an effort to ensure that the entire urethra is filled, the exposure is made while the physician is injecting the contrast medium.

8. True or False. After the bladder is filled with contrast medium, a voiding film can be made with the patient either in a posterior oblique projection or upright.

9. True or False. The radiation field should be large enough to include the entire urinary system on all radiographs.

10. True or False. The image of the urethra should be seen posterior to the superimposed pubic and ischial rami of the dependent side when the patient is properly rotated into a posterior oblique position.

Self-Test: Anatomy and Positioning of the Urinary System

Instructions: Answer the following questions by selecting the best choice.

1. Which renal structure filters the blood?

   a. glomerulus
   b. major calyx
   c. afferent arteriole
   d. efferent arteriole

2. Which urinary excretory duct conveys urine from the bladder to outside the body?

   a. ureter
   b. urethra
   c. afferent arteriole
   d. efferent arteriole

3. Which body organ filters blood and produces urine as a by-product of waste material?

   a. liver
   b. spleen
   c. kidney
   d. pancreas

4. At the level of which vertebra is the superior border of the kidneys usually found?

   a. T10
   b. T12
   c. L2
   d. L4

5. What is the name of the opening on the medial border of a kidney?

   a. pole
   b. base
   c. apex
   d. hilum

6. Which examination is an excretory examination to demonstrate the upper urinary tract?

   a. cystourethrography
   b. retrograde urography
   c. intravenous urography
   d. retrograde cystography

7. Which examination has the ability to produce a radiographic image demonstrating renal cortical tissue well saturated with contrast medium?

   a. cystourethrography
   b. retrograde urography
   c. intravenous urography
   d. retrograde cystography

8. Which renal structures are not demonstrated during a retrograde urographic examination?

   a. ureters
   b. nephrons
   c. minor calyces
   d. major calyces

9. For intravenous urography on a child, what should the patient be given when the scout radiograph shows an excessive amount of intestinal gas overlying the kidneys?

   a. a laxative
   b. a cleansing enema
   c. 12 ounces of iced water
   d. 12 ounces of carbonated beverage

10. Which examination requires the patient to be placed on a special urographic-radiographic examination table?

    a. cystourethrography
    b. retrograde urography
    c. intravenous urography
    d. retrograde cystography

11. In addition to the AP projection, which projection would most likely be included in the radiographs for retrograde urography?

    a. upright AP
    b. recumbent PA
    c. lateral decubitus
    d. posterior oblique

12. What is the purpose of tilting the table 10 to 15 degrees Trendelenburg for retrograde urography?

    a. to demonstrate the ureters
    b. to demonstrate the mobility of the kidneys
    c. to produce a nephrogram effect in the kidneys
    d. to prevent contrast medium from escaping the kidneys

13. **What is the purpose of raising the head of the table 35 to 40 degrees for retrograde urography?**

    a. to demonstrate the ureters
    b. to position the patient for catheterization
    c. to produce a nephrogram effect in the kidneys
    d. to prevent contrast medium from escaping the kidneys

14. Which condition would most likely be demonstrated during voiding cystography?

    a. renal cyst
    b. renal calculi
    c. hydronephrosis
    d. ureteral reflux

15. For the AP projection during retrograde cystography, which procedure should be performed to ensure demonstrating the entire bladder without superimposition with pubic bones?

    a. Direct the central ray perpendicularly.
    b. Angle the central ray 5 degrees caudally.
    c. Angle the central ray 5 degrees cephalically.
    d. Tilt the patient and table 10 to 15 degrees Trendelenburg.

16. For retrograde cystography, which projection/position should be performed to demonstrate anterior and posterior walls of the bladder?

    a. upright AP
    b. recumbent AP
    c. direct lateral
    d. lateral decubitus

17. For cystourethrography with an adult male patient, to what level of the patient should the cassette be centered?

    a. T12 vertebra
    b. L3 vertebra
    c. L5 vertebra
    d. symphysis pubis

18. For cystourethrography with an adult male patient, which projection/position should be used to obtain a radiograph with the patient urinating?

    a. recumbent PA
    b. dorsal decubitus
    c. lateral decubitus
    d. recumbent AP oblique

19. During preparation for intravenous urography (IVU), what is the most likely purpose of obtaining an AP projection radiograph with the patient standing?

    a. to elongate the ureters
    b. to demonstrate ureteral reflux
    c. to demonstrate air-fluid levels
    d. to demonstrate the mobility of the kidneys

20. In intravenous urography (IVU), what is the purpose of applying compression pads over the distal ends of both ureters?

    a. to demonstrate ureteral reflux
    b. to demonstrate the mobility of the kidneys
    c. to retard the excretion of opacified urine from the kidneys
    d. to retard the excretion of opacified urine from the bladder

21. Which of the following is not a reason for obtaining a scout radiograph with the patient recumbent for excretory urography?

    a. to evaluate exposure factors
    b. to demonstrate urinary calculi
    c. to determine the location of the kidneys
    d. to demonstrate the mobility of the kidneys

22. For excretory urography, what should an adult patient do just prior to getting on the examination table?

    a. Remove all jewelry.
    b. Completely empty the bladder.
    c. Drink 12 ounces of iced water.
    d. Drink 12 ounces of carbonated beverage.

23. What is the purpose of obtaining an AP projection radiograph of the kidneys 30 seconds after the bolus injection of a contrast medium in excretory urography?

    a. to demonstrate ureteral reflux
    b. to demonstrate opacified renal cortex
    c. to demonstrate opacified renal arteries
    d. to demonstrate the mobility of the kidneys

24. What is the purpose of tilting the patient and table 15 to 20 degrees Trendelenburg for the AP projection during excretory urography?

    a. to demonstrate distal ureters
    b. to demonstrate opacified renal cortex
    c. to demonstrate the base of the bladder
    d. to demonstrate the mobility of the kidneys

25. How many degrees should the patient be rotated for posterior (AP) oblique projections during excretory urography?

    a. 15
    b. 30
    c. 45
    d. 60

If your school has access to Mosby's Radiographic Instructional Series on Anatomy, Positioning, and Procedures, review Unit 18 at this time; your instructor may request that you respond to the series' exercises on paper. This unit covers the following essential projections:

Urinary system
  AP
  AP oblique, RPO and LPO
  Lateral, R or L
  Lateral, dorsal decubitus
Pelvicalyceal system and ureters
  Retrograde urography
Urinary bladder
  AP and PA
  AP oblique, RPO or LPO
  Lateral, R or L
Male cystourethrography
  AP oblique, RPO or LPO

Chapter 19
REPRODUCTIVE SYSTEM

Part 1

ANATOMY OF THE REPRODUCTIVE SYSTEMS

Exercise 1

Instructions: This exercise pertains to the anatomy of the female reproductive system. Items require you to identify structures, fill in missing words, provide a short answer, or match columns.

1. Identify each lettered structure in Figure 19-1.

A. _____

B. _____

C. _____

D. _____

E. _____

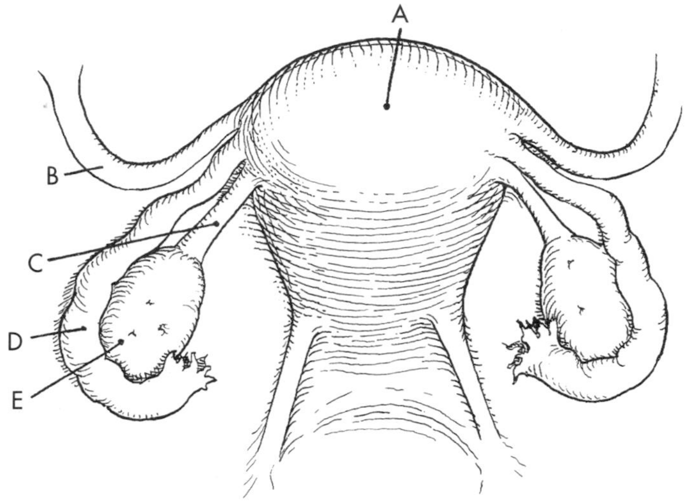

Fig. **19-1.** Superoposterior view of uterus, ovaries, and uterine tubes.

2. Identify each lettered structure in Figure 19-2.

A. _____

B. _____

C. _____

D. _____

E. _____

F. _____

G. _____

H. _____

I. _____

J. _____

K. _____

L. _____

M. _____

N. _____

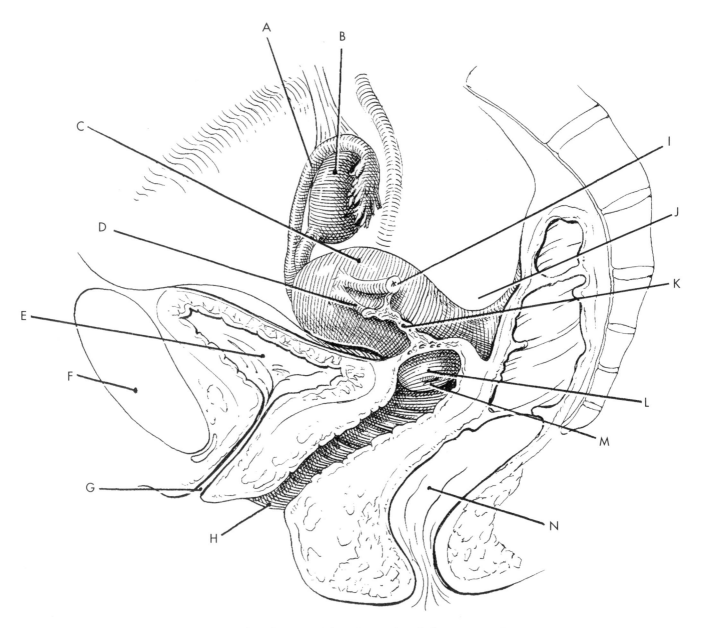

Fig. 19-2. Sagittal section showing relation of internal genitalia to surrounding structures.

3. The female gonads are called the _____.

4. Female reproductive cells are called _____.

5. What structure conveys an ovum from a gonad to the uterus?

6. How many uterine tubes does the typical adult female have?

7. The pear-shaped muscular organ of the female reproductive system is the _____.

8. Name the four main parts of the uterus.

9. Match the uterine structures in Column A with the definitions in Column B.

Column A

____ 1. body

____ 2. fundus

____ 3. cervix

____ 4. isthmus

____ 5. endometrium

Column B

a. superiormost portion

b. cylindrical vaginal end

c. mucosal lining of the uterine cavity

d. constricted area adjacent to the vaginal end

e. where ligaments attach the uterus within the pelvis

10. What part of the uterus is referred to as the *neck?*

Exercise 2

Instructions: This exercise pertains to the anatomy of the male reproductive system. Items require you to identify structures or fill in missing words.

1. Identify each lettered structure in Figure 19-3.

A. _____

B. _____

C. _____

D. _____

E. _____

F. _____

G. _____

H. _____

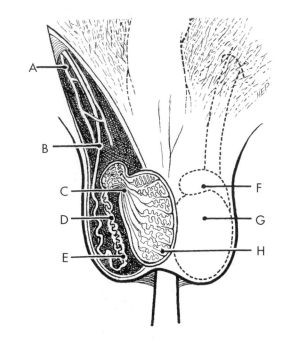

Fig. 19-3. Frontal section of testes and ductus deferens.

2. Identify each lettered structure in Figure 19-4.

A. _____

B. _____

C. _____

D. _____

E. _____

F. _____

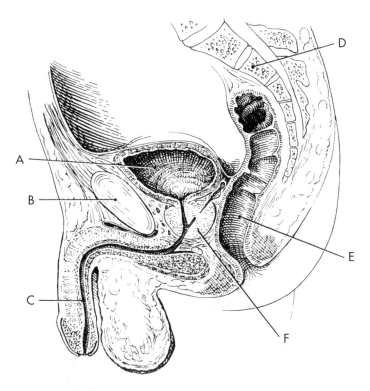

Fig. 19-4. Sagittal section showing male genital system.

3. Identify each lettered structure in Figure 19-5.

A. _____

B. _____

C. _____

D. _____

E. _____

F. _____

G. _____

H. _____

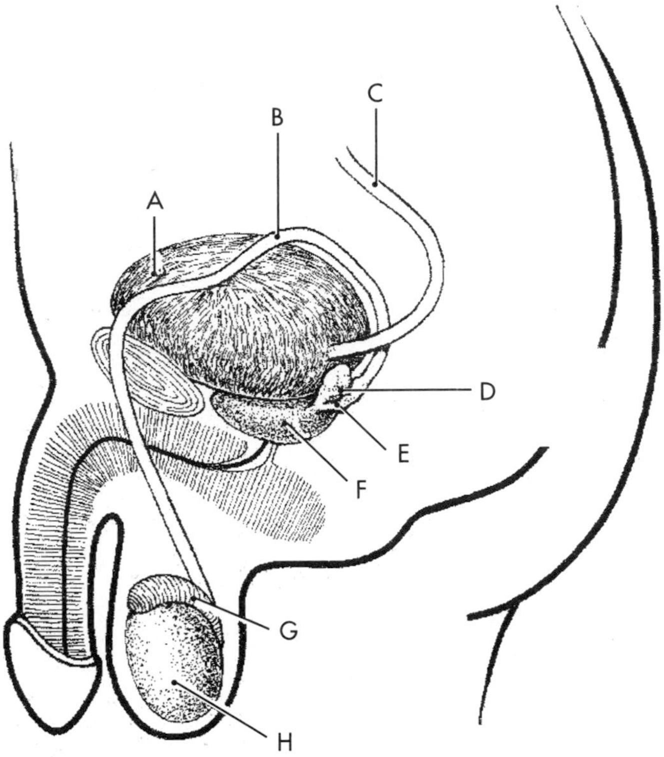

Fig. 19-5. Sagittal section through male pelvis.

4. The male gonads are called the _____.

5. Male reproductive cells are called _____.

6. The oblong structure attached to each testicle is the _____.

7. The excretory channel that allows male germ cells to pass from a gonad to the urethra is the _____

   _____.

8. The union of the ductus deferens and the duct of the seminal vesicle forms the _____ duct.

9. The accessory genital organ that is composed of muscular and glandular tissues is the _____.

10. The ducts from the prostate open into the proximal portion of the _____.

Part 2

RADIOGRAPHY OF THE REPRODUCTIVE SYSTEMS

Exercise 1   Radiography of the Female Reproductive System

Instructions: Although other imaging modalities have reduced the demand for radiographic examinations of the female reproductive system, some facilities still radiographically demonstrate female reproductive structures. This exercise pertains to radiographic visualization of the female reproductive system. Items require you to provide a short answer or match columns.

1. List the three radiographic examinations for the nongravid patient.

2. List the three radiographic examinations for the pregnant patient.

3. Match the descriptions in Column A with the examinations in Column B. Some descriptions may have more than one examination associated with them. Examinations will be used more than once.

Column A

____ 1. determines pelvic diameters

____ 2. uses a Colcher-Sussman ruler

____ 3. helps determine placenta previa

____ 4. requires a gaseous contrast agent

____ 5. requires the use of a contrast agent

____ 6. largely replaced by diagnostic ultrasound

____ 7. performed to demonstrate a fetus in utero

____ 8. investigates the patency of uterine tubes

____ 9. requires a radiopaque contrast agent

____ 10. introduces a contrast agent into the vaginal canal

____ 11. introduces a contrast agent directly into the peritoneal cavity

____ 12. introduces a contrast agent through a uterine cannula

____ 13. should be performed about 10 days after the onset of menstruation

____ 14. performed to determine the size, shape, and position of the uterus and uterine tubes

____ 15. performed to demonstrate congenital abnormalities of the muscular structure that extends from the cervix to the external genitalia

Column B

a. fetography

b. pelvimetry

c. vaginography

d. placentography

e. pelvic pneumography

f. hysterosalpingography

4. Figures 19-6 through 19-10 represent examinations of the female reproductive system. Examine the images, then match the figures in Column A with the examinations in Column B.

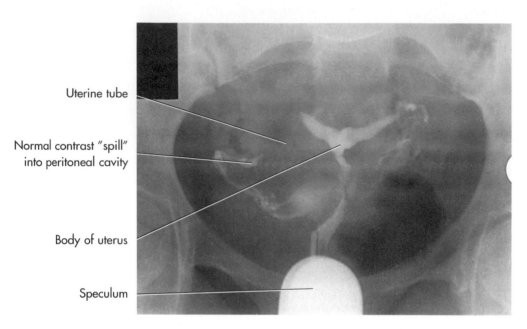

Uterine tube

Normal contrast "spill" into peritoneal cavity

Body of uterus

Speculum

Fig. 19-6. Radiograph of the female reproductive system.

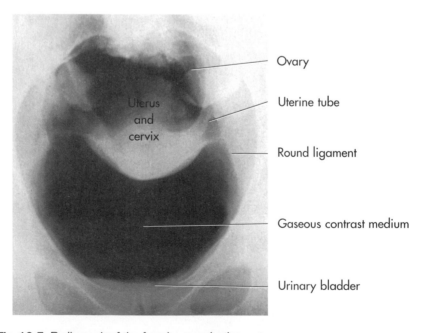

Ovary

Uterine tube

Round ligament

Uterus and cervix

Gaseous contrast medium

Urinary bladder

Fig. 19-7. Radiograph of the female reproductive system.

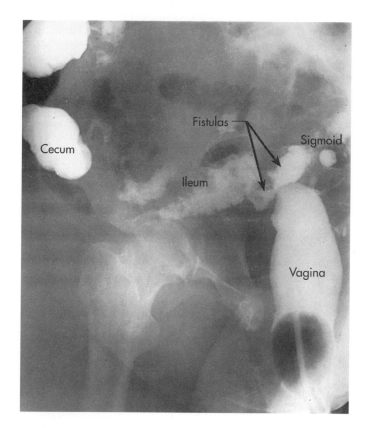

Fig. 19-8. Radiograph of the female reproductive system.

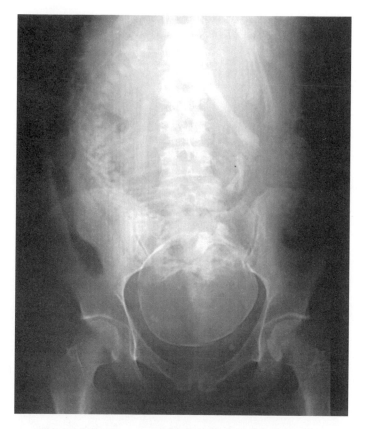

Fig. 19-9. Radiograph of the female reproductive system.

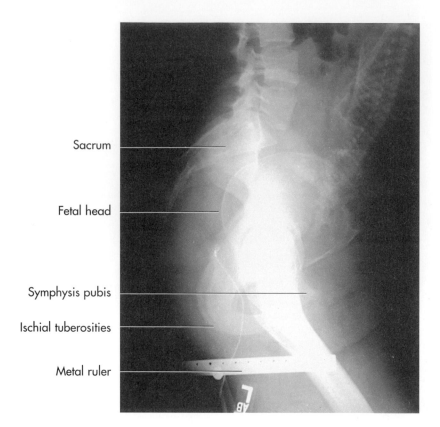

Sacrum

Fetal head

Symphysis pubis

Ischial tuberosities

Metal ruler

Fig. 19-10. Radiograph of the female reproductive system.

Column A	Column B
___ 1. Figure 19-6	a. pelvimetry
___ 2. Figure 19-7	b. fetography
___ 3. Figure 19-8	c. vaginography
___ 4. Figure 19-9	d. pelvic pneumography
___ 5. Figure 19-10	e. hysterosalpingography

Exercise 2 Radiography of the Male Reproductive System

Instructions: The demand for radiographic visualization of the male reproductive system has greatly reduced in recent years because of advances with diagnostic ultrasound; however, some facilities still radiographically demonstrate male reproductive structures. This exercise pertains to radiographic visualization of the male reproductive system. Items require you to provide a short answer.

1. What type of contrast medium is used for radiographic examination of the seminal ducts?

2. For epididymography, why might a radiolucent contrast medium be injected into the scrotum?

3. What accessory organ of the male reproductive system can be radiographically examined?

4. For radiography of the prostate, what body position is preferred? Explain why.

5. For the PA projection of the prostate, how many degrees and in which direction should the central ray be directed?

Self-Test: Reproductive System

Instructions: Answer the following questions by selecting the best choice.

1. Which structures are part of the female reproductive system?

   a. ovaries, uterus, and fallopian tubes
   b. ovaries, testes, and ductus deferens
   c. epididymis, uterus, and fallopian tubes
   d. epididymis, testes, and ductus deferens

2. Which part of the uterus is the most superior portion?

   a. body
   b. fundus
   c. cervix
   d. isthmus

3. Which structure conveys female reproductive cells from a gonad to the uterus?

   a. urethra
   b. uterine tube
   c. ductus deferens
   d. ejaculatory duct

4. Which structure produces female reproductive cells?

   a. ovary
   b. uterus
   c. testicle
   d. epididymis

5. Which structure produces spermatozoa?

   a. ovary
   b. testicle
   c. prostate
   d. epididymis

6. Which structure conveys male reproductive cells from a gonad to the urethra?

   a. uterine tube
   b. fallopian tube
   c. ductus deferens
   d. ejaculatory duct

7. Which structure is attached to each male gonad?

   a. urethra
   b. prostate
   c. epididymis
   d. ejaculatory duct

8. Which examination can be performed on a pregnant patient?

   a. fetography
   b. prostatography
   c. pelvic pneumography
   d. hysterosalpingography

9. Which examination can be performed on a nongravid patient?

   a. fetography
   b. pelvimetry
   c. placentography
   d. hysterosalpingography

10. Which examination introduces contrast medium through a uterine cannula?

    a. fetography
    b. pelvimetry
    c. vaginography
    d. hysterosalpingography

11. Which examination is performed to verify the patency of uterine tubes?

    a. fetography
    b. pelvimetry
    c. placentography
    d. hysterosalpingography

12. Which examination determines pelvic diameters?

    a. fetography
    b. pelvimetry
    c. placentography
    d. hysterosalpingography

13. Which type of contrast medium is preferred for hysterosalpingography?

    a. oily viscous
    b. water-soluble
    c. barium sulfate

14. When should a hysterosalpingographic examination be performed?

    a. after the first trimester
    b. during the first trimester
    c. 10 days after the onset of menstruation
    d. 10 days before the onset of menstruation

15. Which projection is preferred for prostatography?

    a. AP
    b. PA
    c. lateral
    d. lateral decubitus

If your school has access to Mosby's Radiographic Instructional Series on Anatomy, Positioning, and Procedures, review Unit 19 at this time; your instructor may request that you respond to the series' exercises on paper. This unit covers the following examinations:

Female radiography
    Nongravid patient
    Gravid patient
        Fetography
        Radiographic pelvimetry and cephalometry
Pelvimetry
    Localization of intrauterine devices
Male radiography
    Seminal ducts
    Prostate

Chapter 20
SKULL

───── Part 1

OSTEOLOGY OF THE SKULL

Exercise 1

Instructions: This exercise pertains to the osteology of the skull. Items require you to identify structures.

1. Identify each lettered structure in Figure 20-1.

A. _____

B. _____

C. _____

D. _____

E. _____

F. _____

G. _____

H. _____

I. _____

J. _____

K. _____

L. _____

M. _____

N. _____

O. _____

P. _____

Q. _____

R. _____

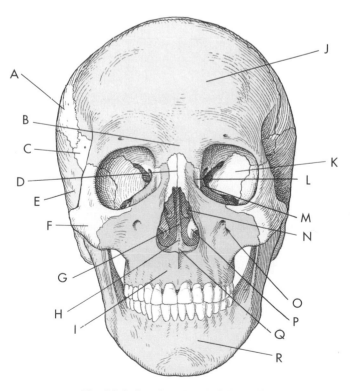

Fig. 20-1. Anterior aspect of the skull.

2. Identify each lettered structure in Figure 20-2.

A. _____

B. _____

C. _____

D. _____

E. _____

F. _____

G. _____

H. _____

I. _____

J. _____

K. _____

L. _____

M. _____ (fontanel)

N. _____ (suture)

O. _____

P. _____ (suture)

Q. _____ (fontanel)

R. _____ (suture)

S. _____

T. _____

U. _____

V. _____

W. _____

X. _____

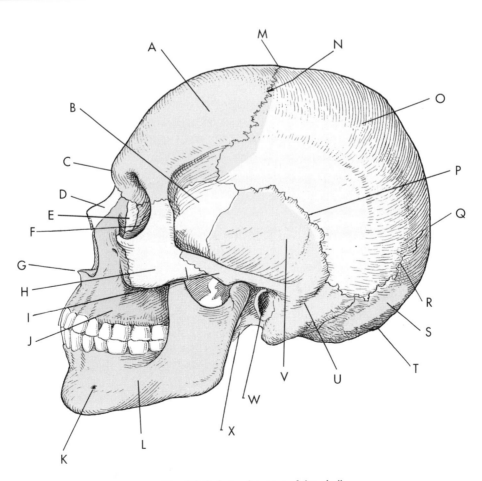

Fig. 20-2. Lateral aspect of the skull.

3. Identify each lettered structure in Figure 20-3.

A. _____

B. _____

C. _____

D. _____

E. _____

F. _____

G. _____

H. _____

I. _____

J. _____

K. _____

L. _____

M. _____

N. _____

O. _____

P. _____

Q. _____

R. _____

S. _____

T. _____

U. _____

V. _____

W. _____

X. _____

Y. _____

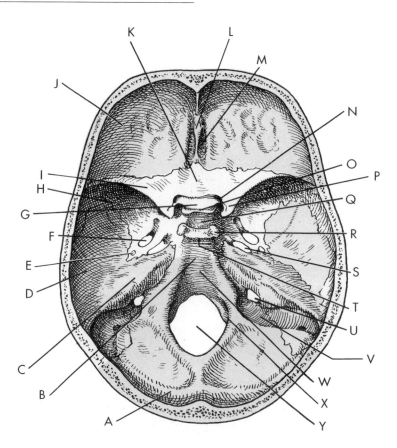

Fig. 20-3. Superior aspect of the cranial base.

4. Identify each lettered structure in Figure 20-4.

A. _____

B. _____

C. _____

D. _____

E. _____

F. _____

G. _____

H. _____

I. _____

J. _____

K. _____

L. _____

M. _____

N. _____

O. _____

P. _____

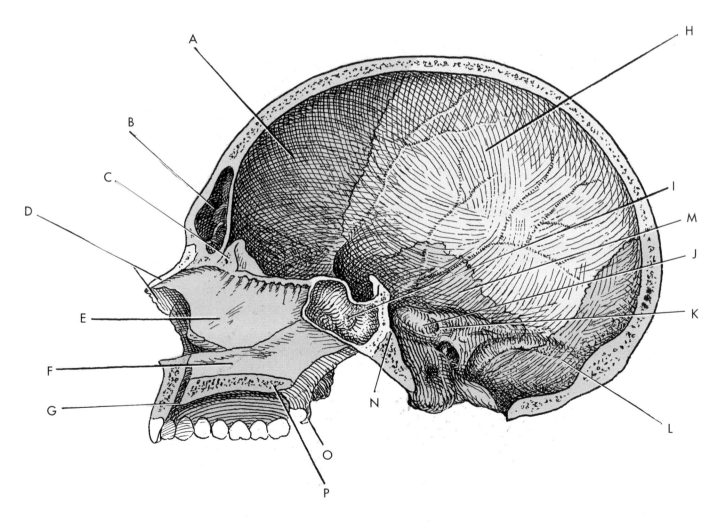

Fig. 20-4. Lateral aspect of interior of the skull.

5. Identify each lettered structure in Figure 20-5.

A. _____

B. _____

C. _____

D. _____

E. _____

F. _____

G. _____

H. _____

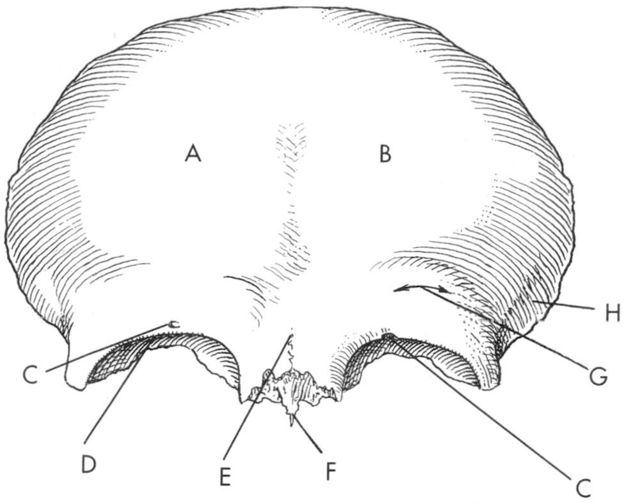

Fig. 20-5. Anterior aspect of the frontal bone.

6. Identify each lettered structure in Figure 20-6.

A. _____   D. _____

B. _____   E. _____

C. _____

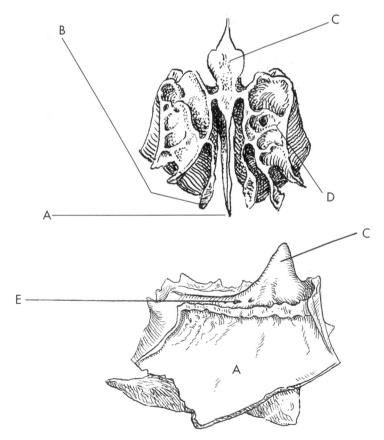

Fig. 20-6. Two illustrations of the ethmoid bone: Diagram **A** shows the anterior aspect; Diagram **B** shows the lateral aspect with the labyrinth removed.

7. Identify the superior border of the parietal bone and each of its four angles in Figure 20-7.

A. _____   D. _____

B. _____   E. _____

C. _____

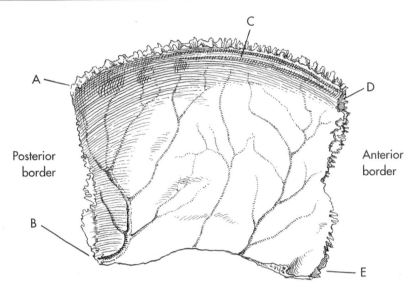

Fig. 20-7. Internal surface of parietal bone.

8. Identify each lettered structure in Figure 20-8.

A. _____

B. _____

C. _____

D. _____

E. _____

F. _____

G. _____

H. _____

I. _____

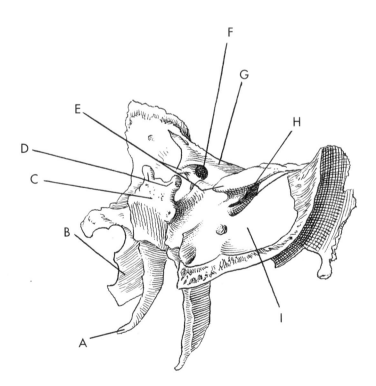

Fig. 20-8. Oblique view of upper and lateroposterior aspects of the sphenoid bone.

9. Identify each lettered structure in Figure 20-9.

A. _____   D. _____

B. _____   E. _____

C. _____

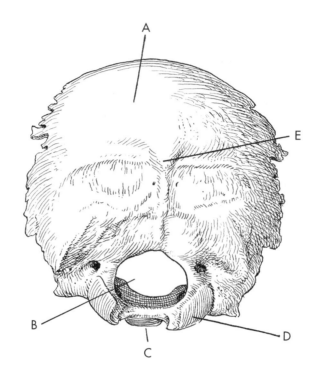

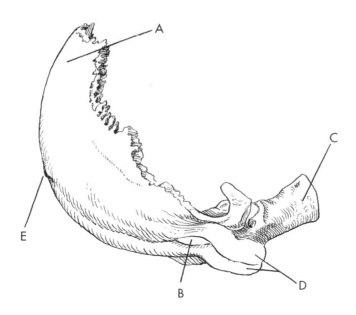

Fig. 20-9. Two illustrations of the occipital bone: Diagram **A** shows the external surface; Diagram **B** shows the lateroinferior surface.

10. Identify each lettered structure in Figure 20-10.

A. _____   F. _____

B. _____   G. _____

C. _____   H. _____

D. _____   I. _____

E. _____

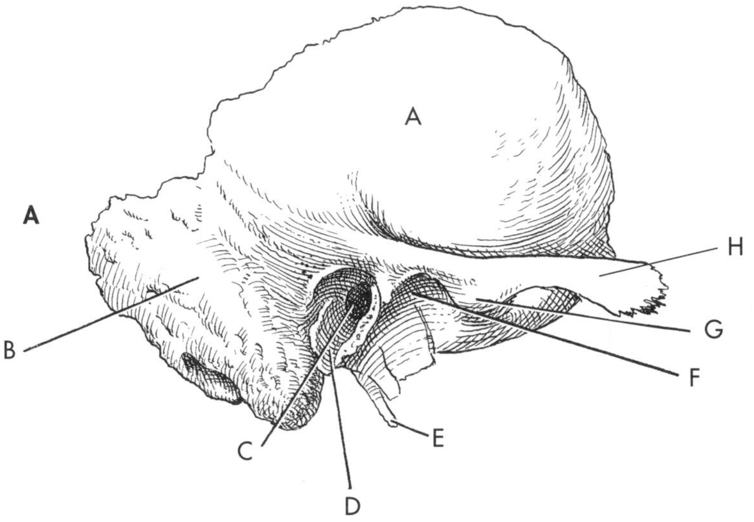

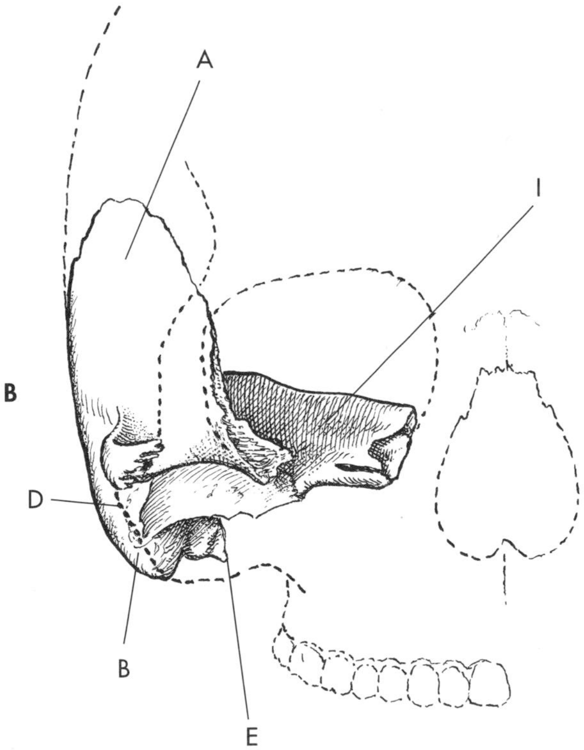

Fig. 20-10. Two illustrations of the temporal bone: Diagram **A** shows the lateral aspect; Diagram **B** shows the anterior aspect in relation to surrounding structures.

11. Identify each lettered structure in Figure 20-11.

A. _____

B. _____

C. _____

D. _____

E. _____

F. _____

G. _____

H. _____

I. _____

J. _____

K. _____

L. _____

M. _____

N. _____

O. _____

P. _____

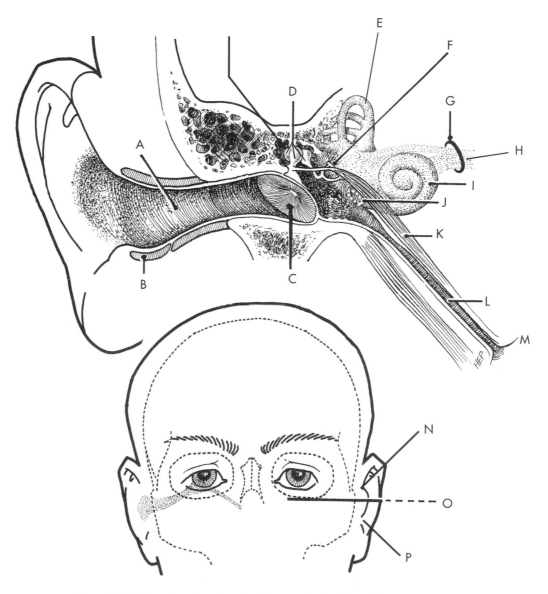

Fig. 20-11. Frontal section through right ear showing internal structures.

12. Identify each lettered structure in Figure 20-12.

A. _____

B. _____

C. _____

D. _____

E. _____

F. _____

G. _____

H. _____

I. _____

J. _____

K. _____

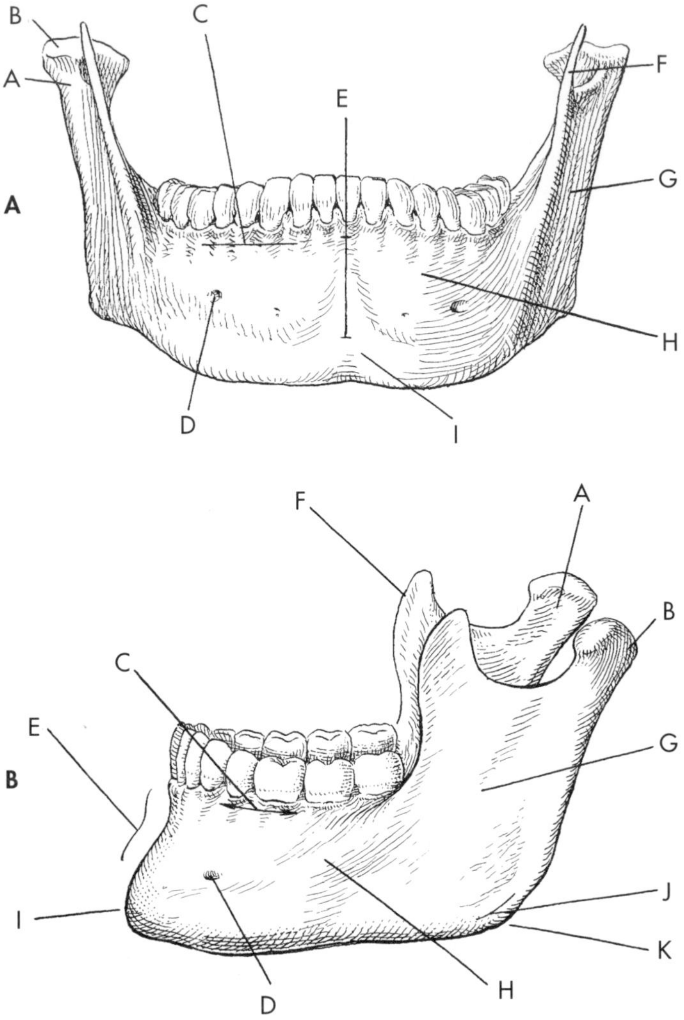

Fig. 20-12. Two illustrations of the mandible: Diagram **A** shows the anterior aspect; Diagram **B** shows the lateral aspect.

13. Identify each lettered structure in Figure 20-13.

A. _____

B. _____

C. _____

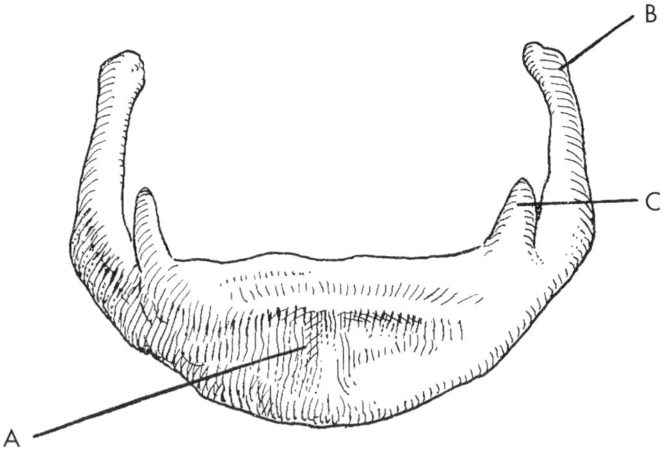

Fig. 20-13. Anterior aspect of hyoid.

Exercise 2

Instructions: Use the following clues to complete the crossword puzzle below. All answers refer to the skull.

ACROSS

1. Perpendicular _____
4. Midpoint of frontonasal suture
5. This bone has wings
7. Vertical part of frontal bone
8. _____ galli
9. Number of cranial bones
12. Densest part of cranial floor
13. Articulates frontal with parietals
16. Synarthrotic cranial joint
19. Anterior fontanel
20. Posterior fontanel
21. Forms top of cranium
22. Posterior part of skull
23. Eyebrow arches

DOWN

1. Inferior sphenoidal process
2. Sphenoidal endocrine
3. _____ turcica
5. Lateral suture
6. Long and narrow skull
10. Average skull
11. Smooth frontal elevation
14. Posterior to nasal bones
15. Ear bone
17. Where occipital joins parietals
18. Forehead bone
19. Anteroinferior occipital part

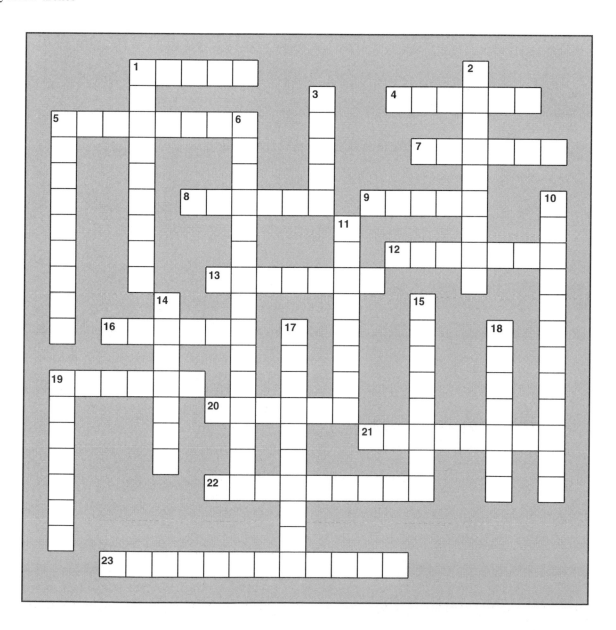

Exercise 3

Instructions: Match the structures in Column A with the cranial bones on which they are found in Column B.

Column A

____ 1. nasion

____ 2. glabella

____ 3. four angles

____ 4. lesser wing

____ 5. greater wing

____ 6. two condyles

____ 7. crista galli

____ 8. sella turcica

____ 9. foramen magnum

____ 10. cribriform plate

____ 11. mastoid process

____ 12. basilar portion

____ 13. petrous portion

____ 14. pterygoid hamulus

____ 15. zygomatic process

____ 16. supraorbital margin

____ 17. perpendicular plate

____ 18. lateral pterygoid process

____ 19. anterior clinoid processes

____ 20. posterior clinoid processes

Column B

a. frontal

b. ethmoid

c. parietal

d. sphenoid

e. temporal

f. occipital

Exercise 4

Instructions: Use the following clues to complete the crossword puzzle below. All answers refer to the facial bones.

ACROSS

2. Another name for zygomatic bone
6. Midpoint of anterior nasal spine
7. Horseshoe-shaped mandibular portion
8. Anterior part of mandibular ramus
10. These have antra of Highmore
12. Articulating process of mandible
14. Serves to attach some throat muscles
15. Vertical mandibular portion

DOWN

1. Found in roof of mouth
3. Found in medial walls of orbits
4. Number of facial bones
5. Cheek bone
9. Spongy processes that hold teeth
10. Largest facial bone
11. Forms inferior portion of nasal septum
12. Extend horizontally inside nasal cavity
13. Forms bridge of the nose

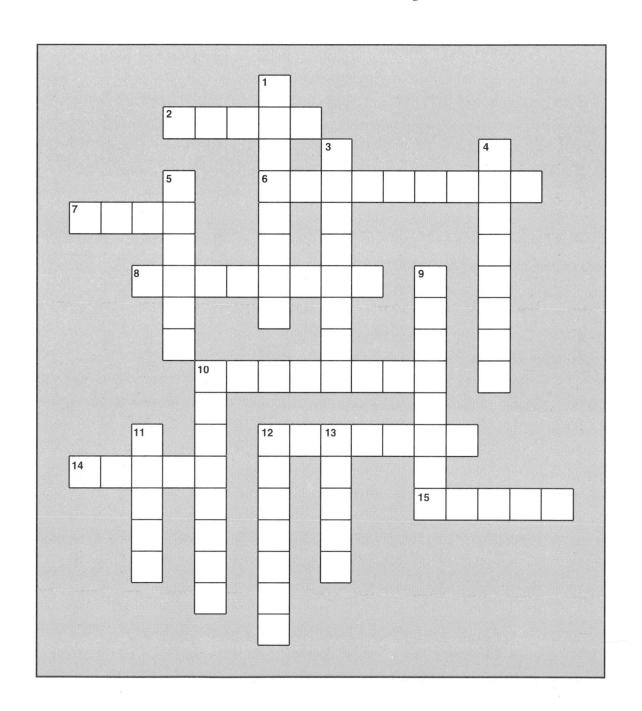

Exercise 5

Instructions: This exercise is a comprehensive review of the osteology and arthrology of the skull. Items require you to fill in missing words or provide a short answer.

1. The bones of the skull are divided into two major groups,

   the _____ bones and the

   _____ bones.

2. List by name and quantity the cranial bones.

3. List by name and quantity the facial bones.

4. The bones of the cranial vault are classified as

   _____ bones.

5. The inner layer of spongy tissue found inside cranial bones

   is called _____.

6. Name the two fontanels located on the median sagittal plane of the skull.

7. What fontanel is located at the junction of the coronal and sagittal sutures?

8. What fontanel is located at the junction of the lambdoidal and sagittal sutures?

9. List the three classifications of fundamental skull shapes, and indicate the number of degrees of angulation formed by the petrous pyramids and the median sagittal plane for each classification.

10. What bone forms the anterior portion of the cranium?

11. What cranial bone is located between the orbits and posterior to the nasal bones?

12. What cranial bones form the vertex and most of the sides of the cranium?

13. The prominent bulge of a parietal bone is called the

    parietal _____.

14. The two parietal bones join together to form the

    _____ suture.

15. The two parietal bones articulate with the frontal bone to

    form the _____ suture.

16. The two parietal bones articulate posteriorly with the

    _____ bone.

17. The two parietal bones and the occipital bone join together

    to form the _____ suture.

18. What cranial bone provides a depression to house the pituitary gland?

19. What cranial bone forms the posteroinferior portion of the cranium?

20. What is the portion of the occipital bone that projects anteriorly from the foramen magnum?

21. What is the name of the large opening of the occipital bone through which part of the medulla oblongata passes?

22. The basilar portion of the occipital bone fuses anteriorly with the body of the _____ bone.

23. With what structure do the occipital condyles articulate?

24. The middle portion of the cranial base is formed by the _____ bone.

25. The organs of hearing are located in the _____ bone.

26. The structure that separates the external acoustic meatus from the auditory ossicles is the _____ membrane.

27. The process of the temporal bone that encloses radiographically significant air cells is the _____ portion.

28. The thickest and densest portion of bone in the cranium is the _____ _____.

29. The petrous portion is a part of the _____ bone.

30. The fibrocartilaginous, oval-shaped portion of the external ear is the _____.

31. Name the three auditory ossicles.

32. The zygomatic process projects anteriorly from the _____ bone.

33. What bone forms part of the cranial base between the greater wings of the sphenoid bone and the occipital bone?

34. What facial bones form the bridge of the nose?

35. The anterior portion of the medial walls of the orbits is formed by the _____ bones.

36. The largest of the immovable bones of the face is the _____ bone.

37. Another name for a maxillary sinus is _____ _____ _____.

38. The thick ridge on the inferior border of the maxillary bone that supports the teeth is the _____ _____.

39. The anterior nasal spine projects superiorly from the _____.

40. The radiographically significant landmark that is the midpoint of the anterior nasal spine is the _____.

41. What facial bones form the inferolateral portion of the orbital margin?

42. What other two names refer to the zygomatic bone?

43. What facial bones form the posterior one-fourth of the roof of the mouth?

44. The scroll-like bony tissues that extend along the lateral

    walls of the nasal cavity are the _____

    _____ _____.

45. What facial bone forms the inferior part of the nasal septum?

46. The largest and densest bone of the face is the

    _____.

47. The portion of the mandible that extends superiorly from

    the posterior aspect of the mandibular body is the

    _____.

48. What is the name of the U-shaped bone located at the base of the tongue?

49. Name the two processes that extend superiorly from a mandibular ramus.

50. What part of the mandible articulates with the mandibular fossa of the temporal bone to form the temporomandibular joint?

──────── Part 2

RADIOGRAPHY OF THE SKULL

Exercise 1 Skull Topography

Instructions: This exercise pertains to positioning landmarks used in skull radiography. Items require you to identify landmarks or provide a short answer.

1. Identify each lettered positioning landmark in Figure 20-14.

A. _____

B. _____

C. _____

D. _____

E. _____

F. _____

G. _____

H. _____

I. _____

J. _____

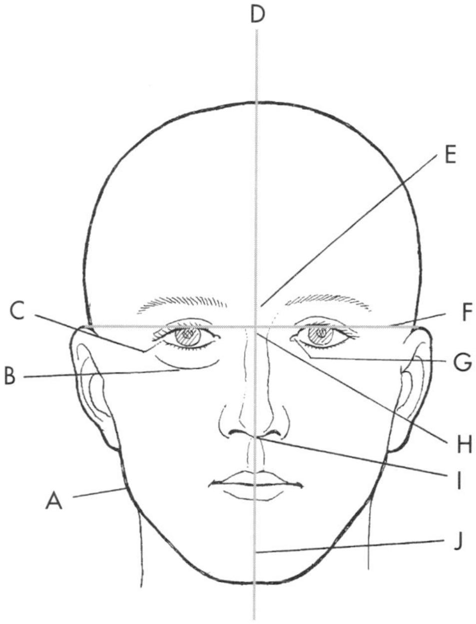

Fig. 20-14. Anterior aspect landmarks.

2. Identify each lettered positioning landmark in Figure 20-15.

A. _____   J. _____

B. _____   K. _____

C. _____

D. _____

E. _____

F. _____

G. _____

H. _____

I. _____

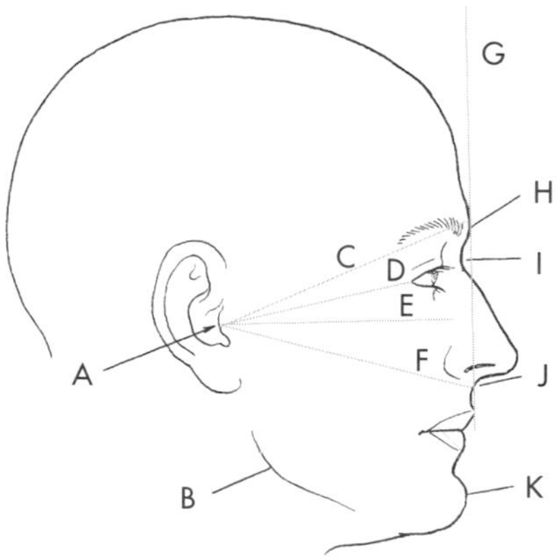

Fig. 20-15. Lateral aspect landmarks.

3. Describe the location of each of the following landmarks on the skull:

a. Inion: _____

b. Vertex: _____

c. Gonion: _____

d. Nasion: _____

e. Glabella: _____

f. Acanthion: _____

g. Mental point: _____

h. Outer canthus: _____

i. Superciliary ridge: _____

4. Name the positioning line of the skull described in each of the following statements:

a. This line extends across the front through both eyes:

b. This line extends from the external acoustic meatus to the outer canthus:

c. This line extends from the external acoustic meatus to the smooth elevation between the superciliary ridges:

d. This line extends from the external acoustic meatus to the inferior margin of the orbit:

e. This line extends from the external acoustic meatus to the midpoint of the anterior nasal spine:

f. This line extends from the glabella to the anterior aspect of the maxilla:

g. This line is also known as the radiographic base line:

h. This line is also known as the base line of the cranium:

i. This plane divides the skull into equal right and left halves:

5. How many degrees of angle difference exist between the following lines?

a. Orbitomeatal and infraorbitomeatal lines: _____

b. Orbitomeatal and glabellomeatal lines: _____

Exercise 2 Positioning for the Cranium

Instructions: The typical radiographic evaluation of the skull, usually referred to as a *skull series,* involves a series of radiographs that may include a PA or AP projection, the AP axial projection, a full basal view, and one or two lateral views. This exercise pertains to those projections. Items require you to identify structures, fill in missing words, provide a short answer, or choose true or false. Explain any statement you believe is false.

Items 1 through 12 pertain to the lateral projection.

1. Indicate how (perpendicular or parallel) the median sagittal plane and the interpupillary line should be positioned with reference to the plane of the film.

a. Median sagittal plane: _____

b. Interpupillary line: _____

2. What positioning line of the head should be parallel with the transverse axis of the film?

3. To what level of the patient should the cassette be centered?

4. What size cassette should be used for the average-size adult skull, and how should it be placed in the cassette holder?

5. Describe how and to where the central ray should be directed.

6. For the cross-table lateral projection with the patient supine, what procedure should be performed to ensure that the entire cranium is included in the image?

7. True or False. For the cross-table lateral projection with the patient supine, the central ray should enter the side of the head at a point 2 inches (5 cm) anterior to the external acoustic meatus.

8. True or False. The temporomandibular joint farther from the film should be demonstrated with superimposition with surrounding structures.

9. List the nine evaluation criteria that indicate the patient was properly positioned for the lateral projection.

10. Figure 20-16 shows two diagrams of a recumbent patient with the median sagittal plane improperly aligned. Examine the diagrams, and explain for each how the position of the patient should be adjusted to properly align the median sagittal plane with the film.

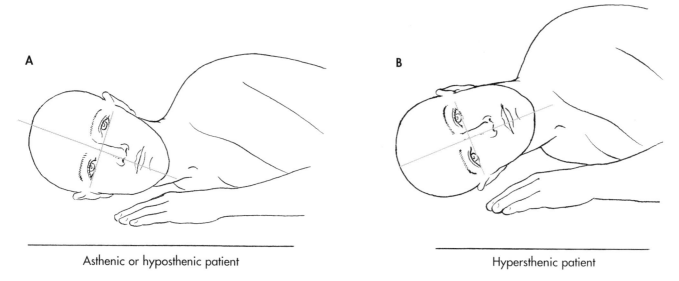

A   B

Asthenic or hyposthenic patient   Hypersthenic patient

Fig. 20-16. Adjusting median sagittal plane with recumbent patient: Diagram **A** refers to asthenic or hyposthenic patient; Diagram **B** refers to hypersthenic patient.

a. Diagram A: _____

b. Diagram B: _____

11. Figures 20-17, 20-18, and 20-19 are lateral projection radiographs of a phantom skull. Only one image demonstrates acceptable positioning. Examine the images and answer the questions that follow. Refer to specific evaluation criteria for this projection when explaining your answers.

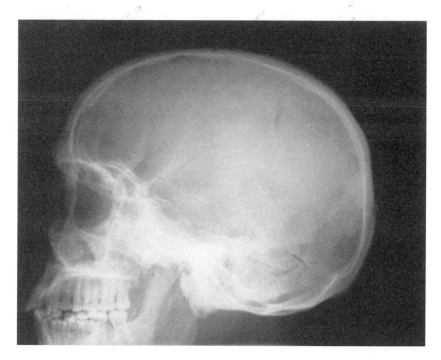

Fig. 20-17. Lateral projection.

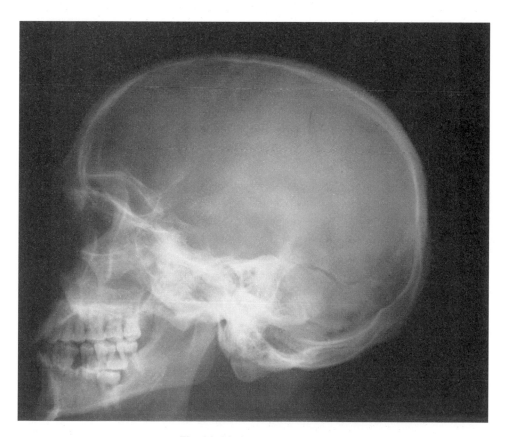

Fig. 20-18. Lateral projection.

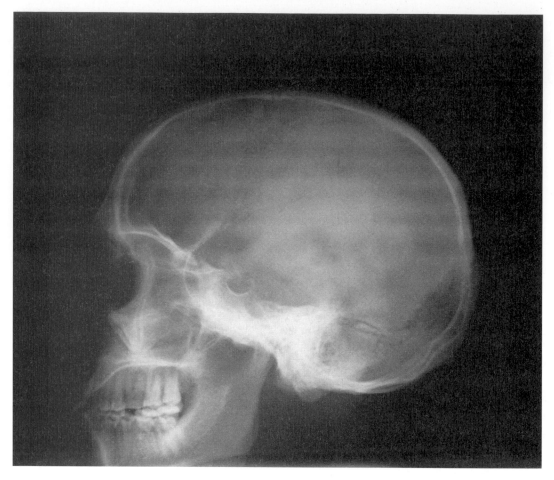

Fig. 20-19. Lateral projection.

a. Which image best demonstrates the skull with optimal positioning? Explain.

b. Which image shows the skull incorrectly positioned because the vertex and median sagittal plane are tilted toward the plane of the film? Explain.

c. Which image shows the skull incorrectly positioned because the face and median sagittal plane are rotated toward the x-ray table and film? Explain.

d. Which image shows the skull positioned similarly to that seen in Figure 20-16, Diagram B?

12. Identify each lettered structure in Figure 20-20.

A. _____   E. _____

B. _____   F. _____

C. _____   G. _____

D. _____   H. _____

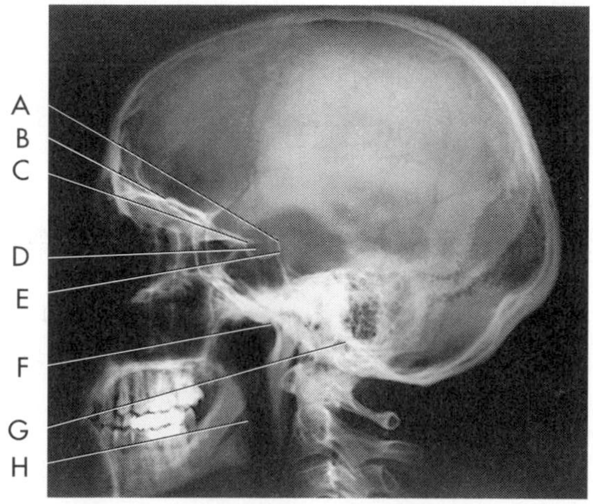

Fig. 20-20. Lateral skull.

Items 13 through 24 pertain to the PA projection, the AP projection, or both.

13. Indicate how (perpendicular or parallel) the median sagittal plane and the orbitomeatal line should be positioned with reference to the plane of the film.

   a. Median sagittal plane: _____

   b. Orbitomeatal line: _____

14. What parts of the patient's facial area should be in contact with the table or vertical grid device?

15. How many degrees and in which direction should the central ray be directed to demonstrate the following structures with the patient positioned for the PA projection of the skull?

   a. Frontal bone: _____

   b. General survey: _____

   c. Superior orbital fissures: _____

   d. Rotundum foramina: _____

16. For the PA projection, the central ray should exit the skull at the _____.

17. The cassette should be centered to the skull at the level of the _____.

18. What breathing instructions should be given to the patient?

19. List the five evaluation criteria that indicate the patient was properly positioned for either the AP or the PA projection.

20. Figure 20-21 shows two AP projection radiographs. Examine each image, and describe how the central ray was directed as well as the specific structures, and their relationship to surrounding structures, that indicate how the central ray was directed.

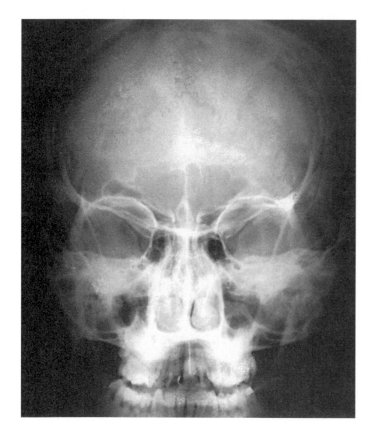
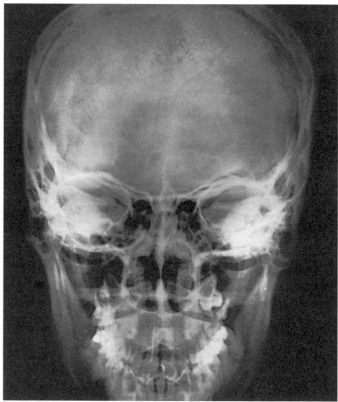

Fig. 20-21. Two views of the AP projection.

a. Diagram A: _____

b. Diagram B: _____

21. Figure 20-22 is a PA projection radiograph of a phantom skull showing incorrect positioning. Examine the image and answer the questions that follow.

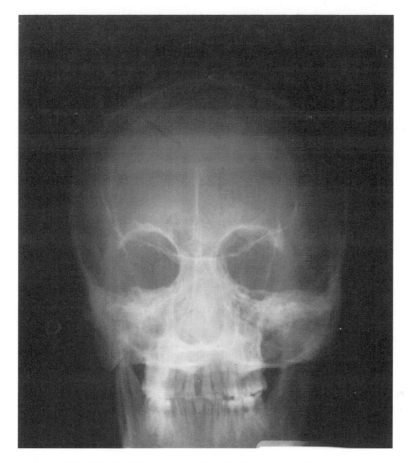

Fig. 20-22. PA projection showing incorrect positioning.

a. Assuming the orbitomeatal line was perpendicular to the plane of the film, describe how the central ray most likely was directed.

b. Describe where the petrous ridges should appear in the image when the central ray is directed caudally 15 degrees.

c. What image characteristic most likely prevents this image from meeting all evaluation criteria for this projection?

d. Describe the positioning error that most likely caused the image to appear as it does.

22. Figure 20-23 is a PA projection radiograph of a phantom skull showing incorrect positioning. Examine the image and answer the questions that follow.

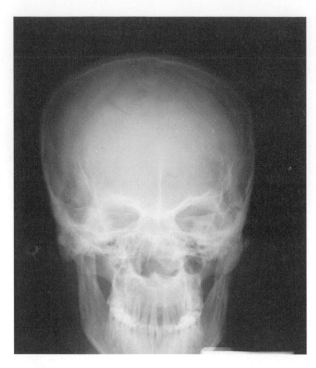

Fig. 20-23. PA projection showing incorrect positioning.

a. Assuming the orbitomeatal line was perpendicular to the plane of the film, describe how the central ray most likely was directed.

b. Describe where the petrous ridges should appear in the image when the central ray is directed caudally 15 degrees.

c. Do the petrous ridges nearly fill the orbits?

d. What image characteristic most likely prevents this image from meeting all evaluation criteria for this projection?

e. Describe the positioning error that most likely caused the image to appear as it does.

23. Figures 20-24 and 20-25 are AP projection radiographs of a phantom skull. Only one image demonstrates acceptable positioning. Examine the images and answer the questions that follow.

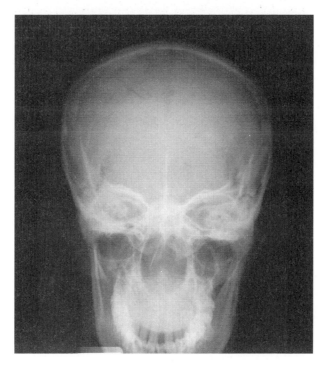

Fig. 20-24. AP projection.

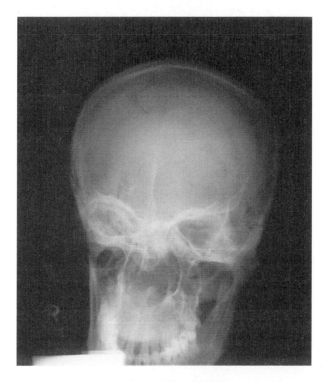

Fig. 20-25. AP projection.

a. Is the positioning quality for Figure 20-24 acceptable or unacceptable?

b. Is the positioning quality for Figure 20-25 acceptable or unacceptable?

c. Describe the positioning error that probably caused the unacceptable image.

d. Assuming that the orbitomeatal line was perpendicular for both images, the central ray appears to have been directed

_____.

24. Identify each lettered structure in Figure 20-26.

A. _____

B. _____

C. _____

D. _____

E. _____

F. _____

G. _____

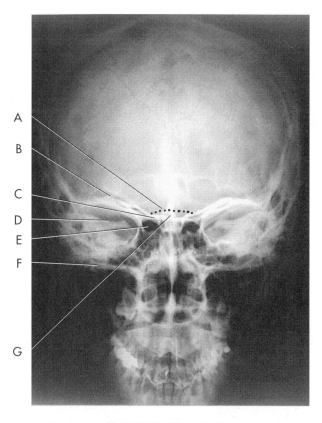

Fig. 20-26. PA projection.

Items 25 through 31 pertain to the AP axial projection (Towne method).

25. The AP axial projection is commonly called the _____ method.

26. To what level of the patient should the upper border of the film be positioned?

27. In addition to the median sagittal plane, either the _____ line or the _____ line must be perpendicular to the plane of the film.

28. What two central ray angulations could be used to properly perform the AP axial projection, and where exactly on the patient's head should the central ray enter?

29. What positioning characteristic determines the number of degrees that the central ray should be angled?

30. List the four evaluation criteria that indicate the patient was properly positioned for the AP axial projection.

31. Identify each lettered structure in Figure 20-27.

A. _____   D. _____

B. _____   E. _____

C. _____   F. _____

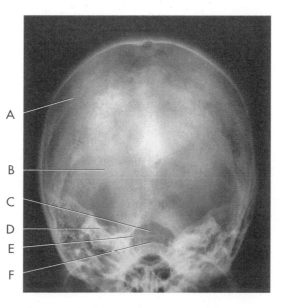

Fig. 20-27. AP axial projection.

Items 32 through 39 pertain to the PA axial projection (Haas method).

32. True or False. The PA axial projection demonstrates the occipital region of the cranium.

33. True or False. Hypersthenic patients should be positioned while recumbent in the supine position.

34. True or False. The PA axial projection (Haas method) is sometimes referred to as the reverse Waters method.

35. In addition to the median sagittal plane, what positioning line of the skull should be perpendicular to the plane of the film?

36. How many degrees and in which direction should the central ray be directed?

37. Where on the skull should the central ray enter?

38. List the four evaluation criteria that indicate the patient was properly positioned for the PA axial projection (Haas method).

39. Identify each lettered structure in Figure 20-28.

A. _____   D. _____

B. _____   E. _____

C. _____

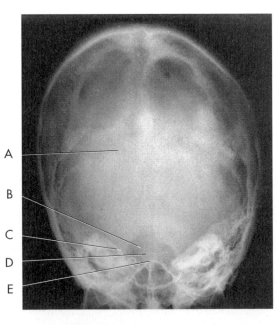

Fig. 20-28. PA axial projection.

Items 40 through 45 pertain to the submentovertical projection.

40. **Indicate how (perpendicular or parallel)** the median sagittal plane and the infraorbitomeatal line should be positioned with reference to the plane of the film.

    a. Median sagittal plane: _____

    b. Infraorbitomeatal line: _____

41. The central ray should be directed perpendicular to the _____ line.

42. Describe where the central ray should enter the patient.

43. List the five evaluation criteria that indicate the patient was properly positioned for the submentovertical projection.

44. Examine Figure 20-29, and state why it does not meet the evaluation criteria for this projection.

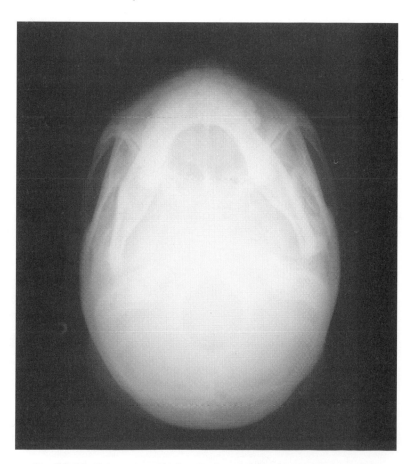

Fig. 20-29. Submentovertical projection showing incorrect positioning.

45. Identify each lettered structure in Figure 20-30.

A. _____

B. _____

C. _____

D. _____

E. _____

F. _____

G. _____

H. _____

I. _____

J. _____

K. _____

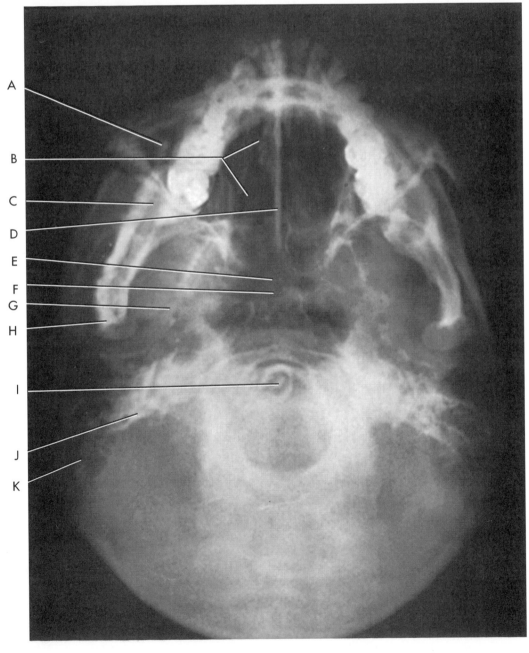

Fig. 20-30. Submentovertical projection.

Exercise 3 Positioning for the Sella Turcica

Instructions: To supplement computed tomography, a tightly collimated image of the sella turcica is often requested. This exercise pertains to the lateral projection of the sella turcica. Items require you to identify structures or provide a short answer.

1. Indicate how (perpendicular or parallel) each of the following should be adjusted to correctly position the patient for the lateral projection of the sella turcica:

   a. Median sagittal plane: _____

   b. Interpupillary line: _____

   c. Infraorbitomeatal line: _____

2. Where on the side of the head should the central ray enter?

3. What breathing instructions should be given to the patient?

4. List the four evaluation criteria that indicate the patient was properly positioned for the lateral projection of the sella turcica.

5. Identify each lettered structure in Figure 20-31.

A. _____   D. _____

B. _____   E. _____

C. _____

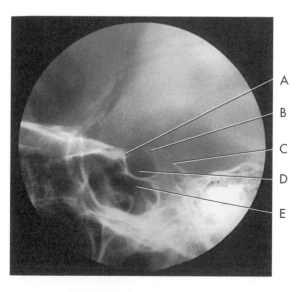

Fig. 20-31. Lateral projection.

Exercise 4 Positioning for the Optic Canal (Foramen)

Instructions: The parieto-orbital oblique projection and the orbitoparietal oblique projection are two standard radiographic procedures used to demonstrate the orbital region, specifically the optic canal. This exercise pertains to those projections. Items require you to identify structures, fill in missing words, provide a short answer, or choose true or false. Explain any statement you believe is false.

Items 1 through 10 pertain to the parieto-orbital oblique projection (Rhese method).

1. What three points of the face should be in contact with the x-ray table or vertical grid device?

2. What positioning line of the head should be perpendicular to the film?

3. The median sagittal plane should form an angle of _____ degrees with the film.

4. True or False. The parieto-orbital oblique projection is considered the PA oblique projection for the orbit.

5. True or False. The affected orbit should be the orbit closer to the film.

6. True or False. The parieto-orbital oblique projection demonstrates a cross-sectional view of the optic canal.

7. True or False. Incorrect angulation of the acanthomeatal line will cause lateral deviation from the preferred location of the optic canal in the imaged orbit.

8. True or False. The central ray should be directed caudally 15 degrees.

9. Figures 20-32, 20-33, and 20-34 are parieto-orbital oblique projection radiographs of a phantom skull. Only one image demonstrates correct rotation of the head. Examine the images and answer the questions that follow. Refer to specific evaluation criteria for this projection when explaining your answers.

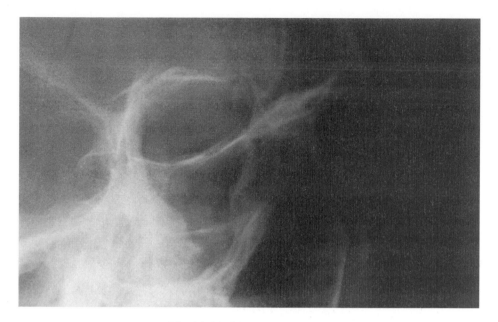

Fig. 20-32. Phantom skull orbit.

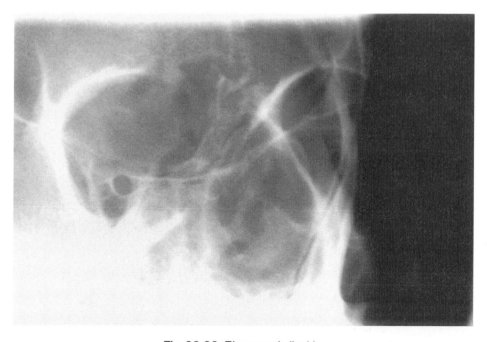

Fig. 20-33. Phantom skull orbit.

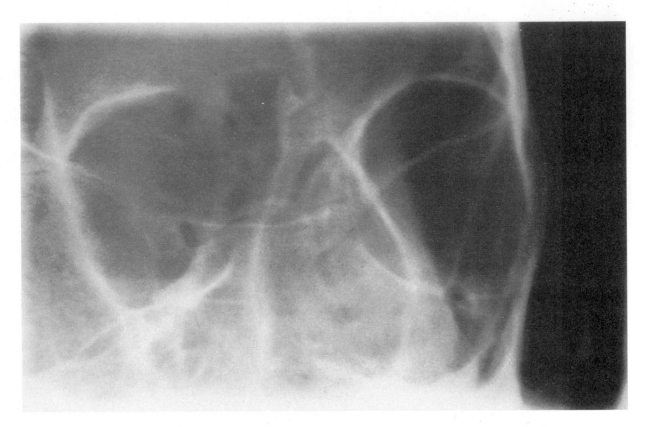

Fig. 20-34. Phantom skull orbit.

a. Which image best demonstrates ideal positioning of the phantom skull? Explain.

b. Which image was made with the median sagittal plane forming an angle with the film considerably less than the required amount? Explain.

c. Which image was made with the median sagittal plane forming an angle with the film somewhat greater than the required amount? Explain.

10. Identify each lettered structure in Figure 20-35.

A. _____   E. _____

B. _____   F. _____

C. _____   G. _____

D. _____

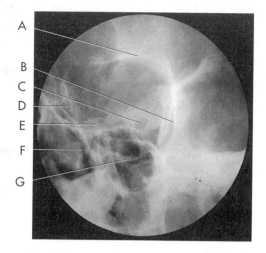

Fig. 20-35. Parieto-orbital oblique projection.

Items 11 through 19 pertain to the orbitoparietal oblique projection (Rhese method).

11. The orbitoparietal oblique projection is considered the reverse of the _____ _____ projection.

12. The patient should be positioned from either the seated-upright position or the _____ (prone or supine) position.

13. True or False. The affected orbit should be the orbit farther from the film.

14. True or False. The orbitoparietal oblique projection causes less radiation exposure to the lens of the eye than does the parieto-orbital oblique projection.

15. True or False. The orbitoparietal oblique projection is considered the PA oblique projection for the orbit.

16. True or False. The orbitoparietal oblique projection results in more magnification of the orbit than does the PA oblique projection.

17. What positioning line of the head should remain perpendicular to the film?

18. What plane should form an angle of 53 degrees with the film?

19. Figure 20-36 is an orbitoparietal oblique projection radiograph of the left orbit of a phantom skull incorrectly aligned. Examine the image and answer the questions that follow.

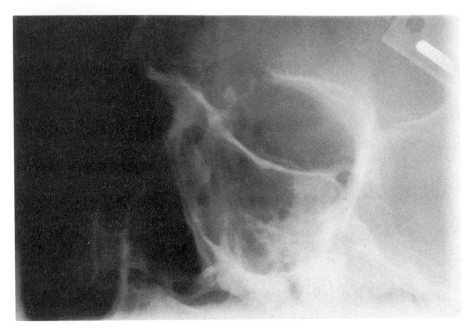

Fig. 20-36. Orbitoparietal oblique projection showing incorrect positioning of a phantom skull.

a. What image characteristic indicates that the phantom skull was not correctly positioned?

b. What positioning error most likely produced this image?

c. How should the patient's position be adjusted to improve the demonstration of orbital structures with a subsequent radiograph?

20. List the four evaluation criteria that indicate the patient was properly positioned for either the parieto-orbital oblique projection or the orbitoparietal oblique projection.

Note to Students: Additional exercises referenced from Chapters 20, 21, 22, and 23 are found in the *Appendix: Supplemental Exercises for Skull Positioning* located in this workbook. Students should complete the review exercises for those chapters before completing the appendix exercises.

If your school has access to Mosby's Radiographic Instructional Series on Anatomy, Positioning, and Procedures, review Unit 20 at this time; your instructor may request that you respond to the series' exercises on paper. This unit covers the following essential projections:

Cranium
    Lateral, R or L
    Lateral (cross-table) R or L
    PA and PA axial, Caldwell method
    AP and AP axial
    AP axial, Towne method
    PA axial, Haas method
Cranial base
    Submentovertical, Schüller method
Sella turcica
    Lateral, R or L
Optic canal: Foramen
    Parieto-orbital oblique, Rhese method
    Orbitoparietal oblique, Rhese method

Chapter 21
FACIAL BONES

Radiography of the Facial Bones

Exercise 1 Positioning for Facial Bones and Nasal Bones

Instructions: A standard radiographic series to demonstrate facial bones includes different projections that examine facial struc-tures from different perspectives. Some projections commonly used are the lateral, the parietoacanthial (Waters method), and the acanthoparietal (reverse Waters method). Additionally, a lateral projection for nasal bones is sometimes added to a facial bones series because nasal bones are sometimes affected when other facial bones are damaged by trauma. This exercise pertains to the projections for facial bones and nasal bones. Items require you to identify structures, fill in missing words, or provide a short answer.

Items 1 through 9 pertain to the lateral projection for facial bones.

1. What plane of the head should be parallel with the film?

2. What positioning line of the head should be perpendicular to the film?

3. What positioning line of the head should be parallel with the upper edge of the film?

4. What facial bone should be centered to the film?

5. What is the purpose of placing a radiolucent pad between the mandible and the x-ray table or vertical grid device?

6. Where on the patient's face should the central ray be directed?

7. List the four evaluation criteria that indicate the patient was properly positioned for the lateral projection for facial bones.

8. Figure 21-1 is a lateral projection radiograph showing incorrect positioning of a phantom skull. Examine the image and state why it does not meet the evaluation criteria for this projection.

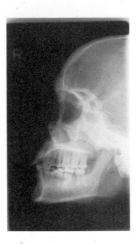

Fig. 21-1. Lateral projection showing incorrect positioning of a phantom skull.

9. Identify each lettered structure in Figure 21-2.

A. _____   E. _____

B. _____   F. _____

C. _____   G. _____

D. _____

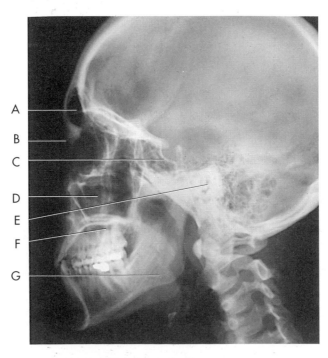

Fig. 21-2. Lateral projection.

Items 10 through 15 pertain to the parietoacanthial projection (Waters method).

10. Indicate how the orbitomeatal line and the median sagittal plane should be positioned with reference to the film.

    a. Orbitomeatal line: _____

    b. Median sagittal plane: _____

11. The cassette should be centered to the patient at the level of the _____.

12. List the two evaluation criteria that indicate the patient was properly positioned for the parietoacanthial projection.

13. Describe where the petrous ridges most likely will appear in the image if the orbitomeatal line produces the following angles with the film:

    a. 25 degrees: _____

    b. 55 degrees: _____

14. Figures 21-3, 21-4, and 21-5 are parietoacanthial projection radiographs of a phantom skull. Only one image demonstrates acceptable positioning. Examine the images and answer the questions that follow.

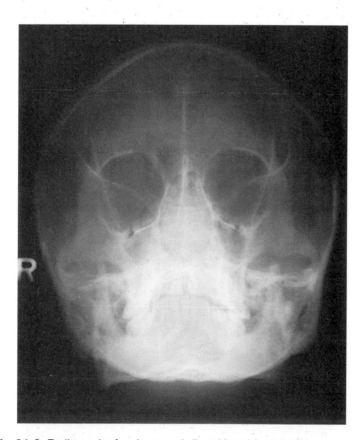

Fig. 21-3. Radiograph of a phantom skull positioned for the parietoacanthial.

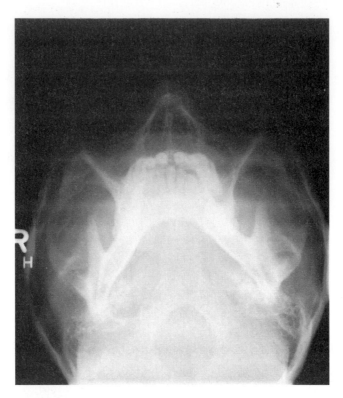

Fig. 21-4. Radiograph of a phantom skull positioned for the parietoacanthial.

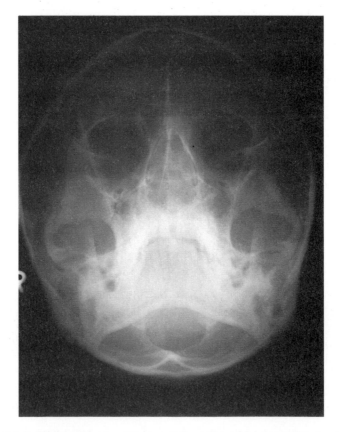

Fig. 21-5. Radiograph of a phantom skull positioned for the parietoacanthial.

a. Which image demonstrates acceptable positioning?

b. In which image does the phantom skull appear to be incorrectly positioned because the angle between the orbitomeatal line and the film is greater than the required amount? (This error results when the patient is unable to extend the neck enough.)

c. In which image does the phantom skull appear to be incorrectly positioned because the angle between the orbitomeatal line and the film is less than the required amount? (This error results when the patient extends the neck too much.)

15. Identify each lettered structure in Figure 21-6.

A. _____   D. _____

B. _____   E. _____

C. _____   F. _____

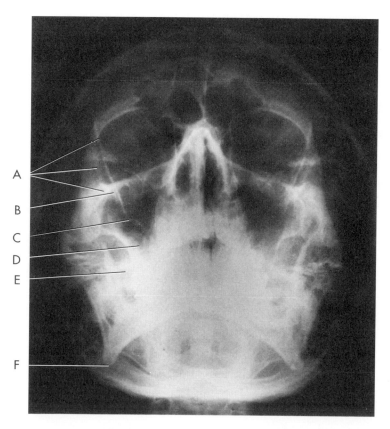

Fig. 21-6. Parietoacanthial projection.

Items 16 through 24 pertain to the acanthoparietal projection (reverse Waters method).

16. The acanthoparietal projection can be used to demonstrate facial bones when the patient is lying in the

_____ position.

17. The image of the acanthoparietal projection is similar to the image of the _____ projection

(_____ method).

18. What two planes or positioning lines of the head should be perpendicular to the film?

19. Where should the midpoint of the cassette be centered to the patient?

20. What breathing instructions should be given to the patient?

21. How many degrees and in which direction should the central ray be directed?

22. The central ray should enter the patient's face at or slightly below the _____.

23. List the two evaluation criteria that indicate the patient was properly positioned for the acanthoparietal projection.

24. Identify each lettered structure in Figure 21-7.

A. _____   C. _____

B. _____   D. _____

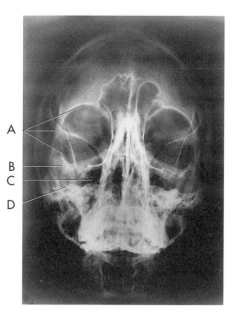

Fig. 21-7. AP axial projection.

Items 25 through 30 pertain to the lateral projection of the nasal bones.

25. Indicate how (perpendicular or parallel) the interpupillary line and median sagittal plane should be positioned with reference to the film.

   a. Interpupillary line: _____

   b. Median sagittal plane: _____

26. How many exposures should be made on one film?

27. The unmasked portion of the film should be centered to the _____.

28. Describe how and to where the central ray should be directed.

29. List the two evaluation criteria that indicate the patient was properly positioned for the lateral projection.

30. Identify each lettered structure in Figure 21-8.

A. _____ (suture)

B. _____

C. _____

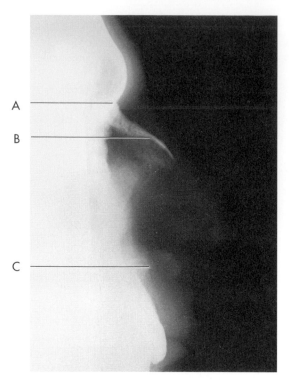

Fig. 21-8. Lateral projection.

Exercise 2 Positioning for Zygomatic Arches

Instructions: Zygomatic arches are commonly demonstrated with three projections: two slightly different tangential projections and the AP axial projection. This exercise pertains to those projections. Items require you to identify structures, fill in missing words, provide a short answer, or choose true or false. Explain any statement you believe is false.

Items 1 through 9 pertain to the tangential (basal) projection.

1. True or False. The tangential (basal) projection should demonstrate both zygomatic arches with one exposure.

2. True or False. Zygomatic arches should be demonstrated superimposed with anterior frontal bone.

3. True or False. The entire cranial base should be demonstrated.

4. True or False. The median sagittal plane should be parallel with the film.

5. What positioning line of the head should be parallel with the film?

6. What projection of the cranium has positioning procedures similar to those of the tangential (basal) projection of the zygomatic arches?

7. Describe how the central ray should be directed.

8. List the three evaluation criteria that indicate the patient was properly positioned for the tangential (basal) projection.

9. Figure 21-9 is a tangential (basal) projection radiograph showing incorrect positioning of a phantom skull. Examine the image and answer the questions that follow.

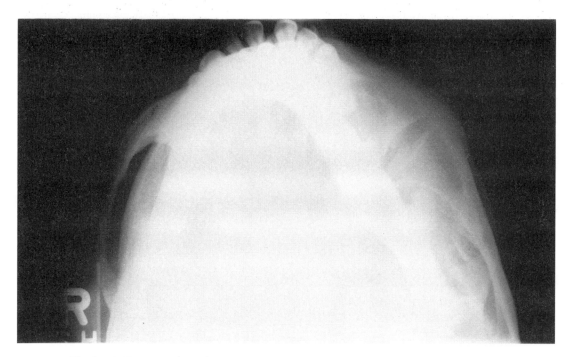

Fig. 21-9. Tangential (basal) projection showing incorrect positioning of a phantom skull.

a. What image characteristics prevent the image from meeting all evaluation criteria for this projection?

b. What positioning error most likely resulted in this unacceptable image?

Items 10 through 14 pertain to the tangential projection.

10. True or False. Both zygomatic arches should be demonstrated on one radiograph with one exposure.

11. True or False. The median sagittal plane should be perpendicular to the film.

12. What positioning line of the head should be parallel with the film?

13. Describe how the central ray should be directed.

14. List the evaluation criterion that indicates the patient was properly positioned for the tangential projection.

Items 15 through 20 pertain to the AP axial projection.

15. Indicate how (perpendicular or parallel) the orbitomeatal line and median sagittal plane should be positioned with reference to the film.

   a. Orbitomeatal line: _____

   b. Median sagittal plane: _____

16. How many degrees and in which direction should the central ray be directed when each of the following positioning lines is placed perpendicular to the plane of the film?

   a. Orbitomeatal line: _____

   b. Infraorbitomeatal line: _____

17. The central ray should enter 1 inch (2.5 cm) above the landmark _____.

18. True or False. Both zygomatic arches should be demonstrated on the radiograph with a single exposure.

19. True or False. The entire vertex should be included on the radiograph.

20. Identify each lettered structure in Figure 21-10.

A. _____

B. _____

C. _____

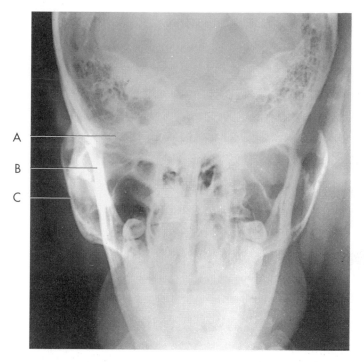

Fig. 21-10. AP axial projection.

Exercise 3 Positioning for the Mandible

Instructions: Usually three or four projections are needed to demonstrate the mandible. The PA, the PA axial, the axiolateral oblique, and the semisupine axiolateral oblique projections are often included in the typical mandible examination. This exercise pertains to those projections. Items require you to identify structures, provide a short answer, or choose true or false. Explain any statement you believe is false.

Items 1 through 10 pertain to the PA projection.

1. What two facial structures should be touching the vertical grid device?

2. What facial structure should be centered to the film for the general demonstration of mandibular rami?

3. How should the median sagittal plane be positioned with reference to the film?

4. What breathing instructions should be given to the patient?

5. Through what positioning landmark of the face should the central ray exit?

6. True or False. The central ray should be directed perpendicularly to the midpoint of the film.

7. True or False. The PA projection demonstrates the mandibular body without bony superimpositioning.

8. List the two evaluation criteria that indicate the patient was properly positioned for the PA projection of the mandibular rami.

9. Figure 21-11 is a PA projection radiograph showing incorrect positioning of a phantom skull. Examine the image and answer the questions that follow.

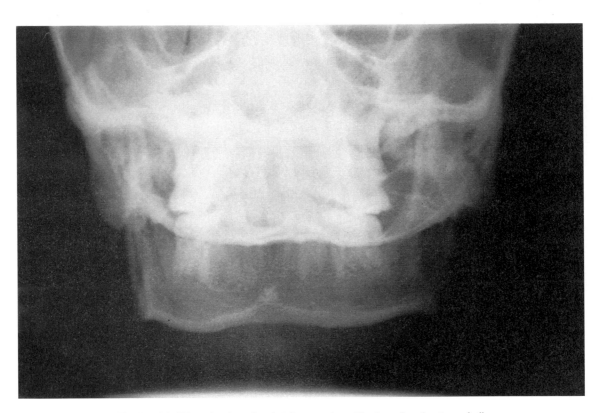

Fig. 21-11. PA projection showing incorrect positioning of a phantom skull.

a. What image characteristic prevents this radiograph from being of acceptable quality?

b. How should the position of the phantom skull be adjusted for a subsequent radiograph?

10. Identify each lettered structure and fracture in Figure 21-12.

A. _____   C. _____

B. _____   D. _____

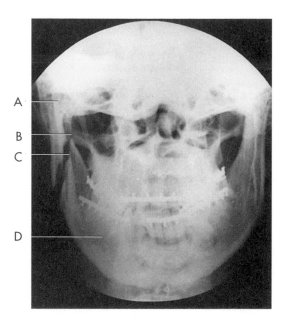

Fig. 21-12. PA projection.

Items 11 through 17 pertain to the PA axial projection.

11. What two facial structures should be touching the vertical grid device?

12. What positioning landmark should be centered to the film to demonstrate the condylar processes?

13. How should the median sagittal plane be positioned with reference to the film?

14. What breathing instructions should be given to the patient?

15. For the PA axial projection to demonstrate the condylar processes, how many degrees and in which direction should the central ray be directed?

16. What prevents the central part of the mandibular body from being clearly demonstrated with the PA axial projection?

17. List the three evaluation criteria that indicate the patient was properly positioned for the PA axial projection.

Items 18 through 26 pertain to the axiolateral oblique projection performed with the patient prone or upright.

18. True or False. The head should be placed in a true lateral position.

19. True or False. The central ray should be directed 15 degrees caudad.

20. What major part of the mandible is demonstrated with the axiolateral oblique projection?

21. Describe where the central ray should enter the patient.

22. Describe how the patient's head should be adjusted.

23. What part of the mandible should be parallel with the film?

24. List the two evaluation criteria that indicate the patient was properly positioned for the axiolateral oblique projection.

25. Figure 21-13 is **an axiolateral oblique** projection radiograph showing incorrect positioning of a phantom skull. Examine the image and answer the questions that follow.

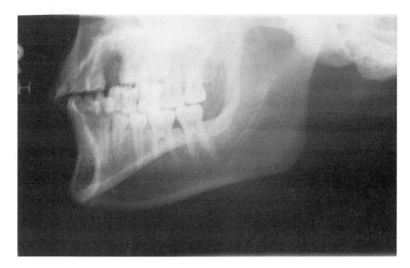

Fig. 21-13. Axiolateral oblique projection showing incorrect positioning of a phantom skull.

a. What image characteristic prevents the image from meeting all evaluation criteria for this projection?

b. How should the position of the phantom skull be adjusted for a subsequent radiograph?

26. Identify each lettered structure in Figure 21-14.

A. _____

B. _____

C. _____

D. _____

E. _____

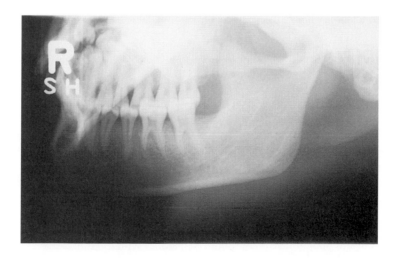

Fig. 21-14. Axiolateral oblique projection.

Items 27 through 35 pertain to the axiolateral oblique (semisupine) projection.

27. True or False. The patient should be placed in a semisupine position with the affected side down.

28. True or False. The head should be adjusted in a true AP position.

29. True or False. In the image of the semisupine axiolateral oblique projection, the central part of the mandibular body is not well seen because of the superimposed spine.

30. True or False. The cassette should be placed on a support to cause it to be cranially inclined with the edge nearest the shoulder elevated.

31. True or False. The long axis of the mandibular body should be positioned parallel with the transverse axis of the film.

32. How many degrees and in which direction should the central ray be directed?

33. Where should the central ray enter the patient?

34. What breathing instructions should be given to the patient?

35. Indicate on what part of the facial area the head should rest to demonstrate the following mandibular areas:

   a. Anterior one-third of the body: _____

   b. Posterior two-thirds of the body: _____

Exercise 4 Positioning for the Temporomandibular Joints

Instructions: Two projections often performed to demonstrate temporomandibular joints (TMJs) are the AP axial projection and the axiolateral oblique projection. This exercise pertains to those projections. Items require you to identify structures, provide a short answer, or choose true or false. Explain any statement you believe is false.

Items 1 through 10 pertain to the AP axial projection.

 1. True or False. For the AP axial projection in the closed-mouth position, the upper posterior teeth should be in contact with the lower posterior teeth.

 2. True or False. The long axis of the mandibular body should be parallel with the transverse axis of the film.

3. Why should the incisors not be occluded when the patient is positioned for the closed-mouth AP axial projection?

4. Identify a situation in which the patient should not be asked to open the mouth wide for the AP axial projection. Explain why.

5. What plane and positioning line of the head should be perpendicular to the film?

6. To what level of the patient should the cassette be centered?

7. How many degrees and in which direction should the central ray be directed?

8. Where should the central ray enter the patient?

9. List the two evaluation criteria that indicate the patient was properly positioned for the AP axial projection with the mouth closed.

10. List the two evaluation criteria that indicate the patient was properly positioned for the AP axial projection with the mouth open.

Items 11 through 20 pertain to the axiolateral oblique projection.

11. How should the median sagittal plane be positioned with reference to the film?

12. What positioning line of the head should be parallel with the transverse axis of the film?

13. Where on the patient should the cassette be centered?

14. How many degrees and in which direction should the central ray be directed?

15. True or False. The central ray should enter the patient at the TMJ farther from the film.

16. True or False. Both open- and closed-mouth positions should be performed with the axiolateral oblique projection unless contraindicated.

17. True or False. The entire side of the mandible from the condyle to the symphysis should be demonstrated.

18. In relation to surrounding structures, where in the image should the mandibular condyle be seen for the axiolateral oblique projection with the patient holding the mouth closed?

19. Through what structure should the central ray exit the patient?

20. Identify each lettered structure in Figure 21-15.

A. _____   C. _____

B. _____

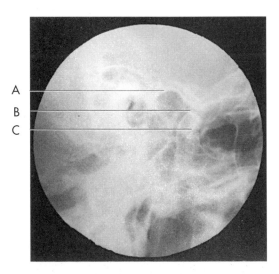

Fig. 21-15. Axiolateral oblique projection with the patient's mouth open.

Note to Students: Additional exercises referenced from Chapters 20, 21, 22, and 23 are found in the *Appendix: Supplemental Exercises for Skull Positioning* located in this workbook. Students should complete the review exercises for those chapters before completing the appendix exercises.

If your school has access to Mosby's Radiographic Instructional Series on Anatomy, Positioning, and Procedures, review Unit 21 at this time; your instructor may request that you respond to the series' exercises on paper. This unit covers the following essential projections:

Facial bones
    Lateral, R or L
    Parietoacanthial, Waters method
    Acanthoparietal, reverse Waters method
Nasal bones
    Lateral, R and L
Zygomatic arches
    Tangential
    Tangential (single arch)
    AP axial
Mandibular rami
    PA
    PA axial
Mandible
    Axiolateral oblique (prone)
    Axiolateral oblique (semisupine)
Temporomandibular articulations
    AP axial
    Axiolateral oblique, R and L

Chapter 22
PARANASAL SINUSES

Chapter 22 Review

Instructions: Usually three or four of the following projections comprise the typical paranasal sinus series: the lateral, the PA axial (Caldwell method), the parietoacanthial (Waters method), the submentovertical (basal), and the PA. This exercise pertains to the paranasal sinuses and the projections used to demonstrate them. Items require you to identify structures, fill in missing words, provide a short answer, or choose true or false. Explain any statement you believe is false.

Items 1 through 10 pertain to the sinuses and radiographic procedures for the sinuses.

1. Name the four groups of sinuses.

2. Identify each lettered structure in Figure 22-1.

A. _____   C. _____

B. _____   D. _____

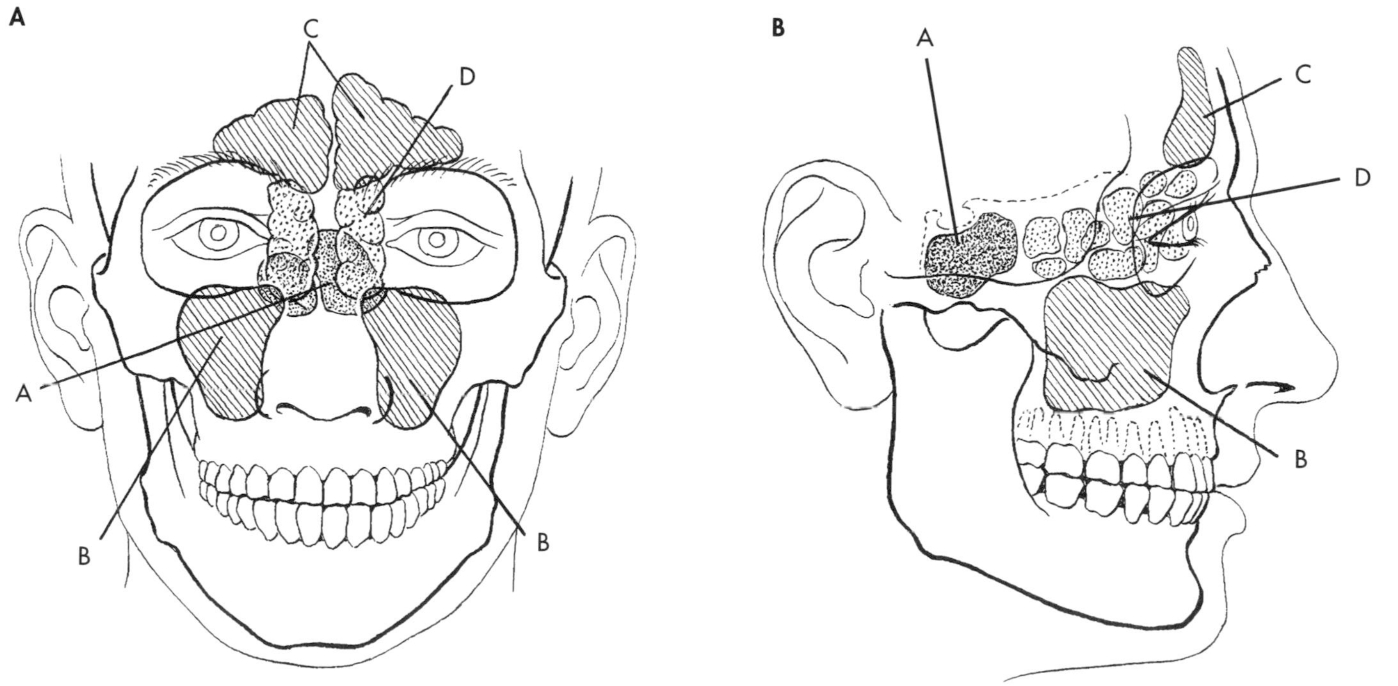

Fig. 22-1. Two diagrams showing paranasal sinuses in relation to each other and surrounding structures: Diagram **A** shows the frontal view; Diagram **B** shows a lateral view.

3. What paranasal sinus group is located more superiorly than the other sinus groups?

4. What paranasal sinuses are also referred to as the antra of Highmore?

5. What paranasal sinuses are located directly below the sella turcica?

6. What paranasal sinus group is located posterior to the ethmoidal sinuses?

7. The ethmoidal sinuses are subdivided into three main groups: the _____ air cells, the

   _____ air cells, and the _____ air cells.

8. Routinely, the paranasal sinuses should be radiographed with the patient in the _____ position.

9. Give two reasons that the patient should be positioned as indicated in item 8.

10. Why should the radiographer ensure that the exposure factors used do not cause the paranasal sinuses to appear underpenetrated?

Items 11 through 17 pertain to the lateral projection.

11. The lateral projection for paranasal sinuses is similar to the lateral projection for the cranium because the

    _____ _____ plane should be _____ with the film.

12. The lateral projection for paranasal sinuses is similar to the lateral projection for the cranium because the

    _____ line should be _____ to the film.

13. What location on the patient's head should be centered to the film?

14. What sinus group is of primary importance?

15. How many sinus groups are usually demonstrated with the lateral projection radiograph?

16. List the six evaluation criteria that indicate the patient was properly positioned for the lateral projection.

17. Identify each lettered structure in Figure 22-2.

A. _____   D. _____

B. _____   E. _____

C. _____   F. _____

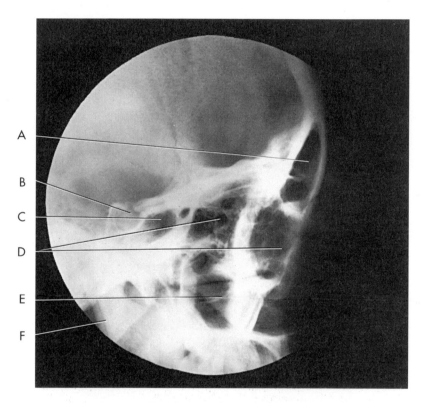

Fig. 22-2. Lateral projection.

Items 18 through 25 pertain to the PA axial projection (Caldwell method).

18. What positioning line should be perpendicular to the film for each Caldwell method?

　a. Original Caldwell: _____

　b. Modified Caldwell: _____

19. How many degrees and in which direction should the central ray be directed for each Caldwell method?

　a. Original Caldwell: _____

　b. Modified Caldwell: _____

20. How should the vertical grid device be adjusted when a horizontal central ray is directed to the patient?

21. To what positioning landmark of the skull should the film be centered?

22. This projection primarily demonstrates the _____ sinuses and the _____

     _____ air cells.

23. Where should the petrous ridges be demonstrated in the image?

24. List the six evaluation criteria that indicate the patient was properly positioned for the PA axial projection.

25. Identify each lettered structure in Figure 22-3.

A. _____   D. _____

B. _____   E. _____

C. _____   F. _____

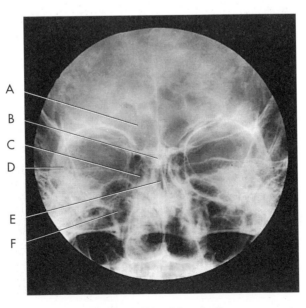

Fig. 22-3. PA axial projection.

Items 26 through 37 pertain to the parietoacanthial projection (Waters method).

26. What paranasal sinuses are best demonstrated with the parietoacanthial projection (Waters method)?

27. What major paranasal sinus group is not seen in the image?

28. Where should petrous ridges be demonstrated in the image?

29. Where will the petrous ridges be demonstrated in the image if the patient does not sufficiently extend the neck?

30. How will the maxillary sinuses appear in the image if the patient extends the neck too much?

31. True or False. The patient's nose and forehead should touch the vertical grid device.

32. True or False. The median sagittal plane should be perpendicular to the film.

33. What positioning line of the head should form an angle of 37 degrees with the film?

34. The cassette should be centered to the _____.

35. The open-mouth modification demonstrates the _____ sinuses through the patient's mouth.

36. List the six evaluation criteria that indicate the patient was properly positioned for the parietoacanthial projection (Waters method).

37. Identify each lettered structure in Figure 22-4.

A. _____   D. _____

B. _____   E. _____

C. _____   F. _____

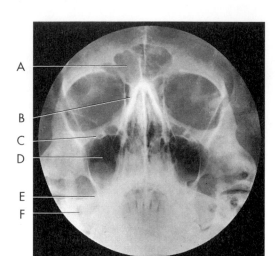

Fig. 22-4. Parietoacanthial projection.

Items 38 through 50 pertain to the submentovertical (basal) projection.

38. True or False. The median sagittal plane should be perpendicular to the film.

39. True or False. The orbitomeatal line should be as nearly parallel with the film as possible.

40. True or False. The central ray should be directed perpendicularly, entering the midline of the base of the skull so that it passes through the sphenoidal sinus.

41. True or False. Close collimation of the x-ray beam should include the anterior cranial base.

42. True or False. The distance from the lateral border of the skull to the lateral border of the mandibular condyles should be the same on both sides.

43. True or False. The entire occipital bone should be included in the image of the submentovertical projection to demonstrate paranasal sinuses.

44. How will the image of the submentovertical projection appear if the position of the median sagittal plane is sufficiently tilted to prevent it from being perpendicular to the film?

45. What two sinus groups are well demonstrated with the submentovertical projection?

46. Where in the image should the mandibular symphysis appear in relation to the frontal bone?

47. What positioning error most likely occurred if the mandibular symphysis is imaged posterior to, and separated from, the anterior frontal bone?

48. What positioning error most likely occurred if the mandibular symphysis is imaged superior to the anterior frontal bone?

49. Where in the image should the mandibular condyles appear in relation to surrounding structures?

50. Identify each lettered structure in Figure 22-5.

A. _____

B. _____

C. _____

D. _____

E. _____

F. _____

G. _____

H. _____

I. _____

J. _____

K. _____

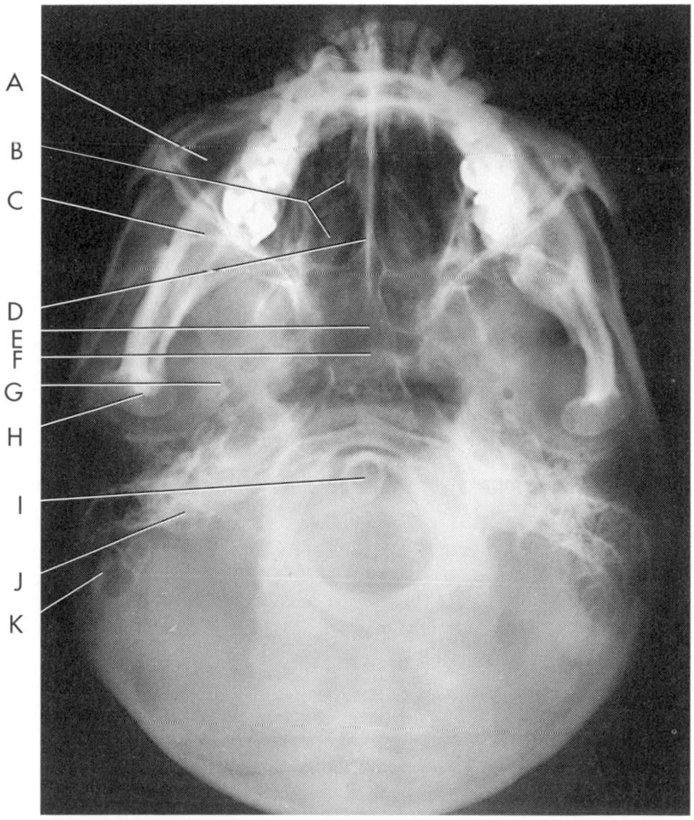

Fig. 22-5. Submentovertical projection.

Items 51 through 60 pertain to the PA projections.

51. True or False. The PA projection requires the median sagittal plane to be perpendicular to the film.

52. True or False. The patient should be placed in the upright position.

53. True or False. The entire cranium should be included in the image for each PA projection for sinuses.

54. True or False. The patient should be requested to breathe slowly during the exposure to produce a suitable background density with which to better demonstrate maxillary sinuses.

55. What positioning line of the head should be perpendicular to the plane of the film?

56. Describe how and to where the central ray should be directed for the PA projection to demonstrate the following sinus groups:

    a. Posterior ethmoidal sinuses: _____

    b. Sphenoidal sinuses: _____

    c. Maxillary sinuses: _____

57. Describe in relation to surrounding structures where the posterior ethmoidal sinuses should be seen in the image.

58. Describe in relation to surrounding structures where the sphenoidal sinuses should be seen in the image.

59. Describe in relation to surrounding structures where the maxillary sinuses should be seen in the image.

60. Identify the three evaluation criteria that indicate the patient was properly positioned for all three PA projections for sinuses.

Note to Students: Additional exercises referenced from Chapters 20, 21, 22, and 23 are found in the *Appendix: Supplemental Exercises for Skull Positioning* located in this workbook. Students should complete the review exercises for those chapters before completing the appendix exercises.

If your school has access to Mosby's Radiographic Instructional Series on Anatomy, Positioning, and Procedures, review Unit 22 at this time; your instructor may request that you respond to the series' exercises on paper. This unit covers the following essential projections:

Paranasal sinuses
  Lateral, R or L
Frontal and anterior ethmoidal sinuses
  PA axial, Caldwell method
Maxillary sinuses
  Parietoacanthial, Waters method (with open-
    mouth modification)
Ethmoidal and sphenoidal sinuses
  Submentovertical
  Ethmoidal, sphenoidal, and maxillary sinuses
  PA

Chapter 23
TEMPORAL BONE

Chapter 23 Review

Instructions: Although computed tomography is often used to image internal cranial structures, standard radiography is still employed in small medical facilities to demonstrate mastoid processes and petrous portions. An axiolateral projection (Law method) can be used to image mastoid air cells, and both axiolateral oblique projections (posterior profile [Stenvers method] and anterior profile [Arcelin method]) can demonstrate petrous portions. This exercise pertains to those projections. Items require you to identify structures, fill in missing words, provide a short answer, or choose true or false. Explain any statement you believe is false.

Items 1 through 11 pertain to the axiolateral projection (Law method; single tube-angulation method).

1. True or False. The patient's head should be placed and maintained in the true lateral position.

2. True or False. The patient's head should be rotated from the true AP position until the median sagittal plane forms an angle of 15 degrees from vertical.

3. True or False. The interpupillary line should remain perpendicular to the film throughout the positioning procedure.

4. Describe how the patient's head should be positioned.

5. What procedure should be performed to prevent soft-tissue structures from overlapping the mastoid process of interest?

6. If the patient is rotated 15 degrees from the right lateral position, what mastoid process is of interest? Is it the side closer to or farther from the film?

7. Where should the cassette be centered to the patient?

8. How many degrees and in which direction should the central ray be directed?

9. Where should the central ray enter the patient?

10. List the six evaluation criteria that indicate the patient was properly positioned for the single tube-angulation method for the axiolateral projection (Law method).

11. Identify each lettered structure in Figure 23-1.

A. _____   D. _____

B. _____   E. _____

C. _____   F. _____

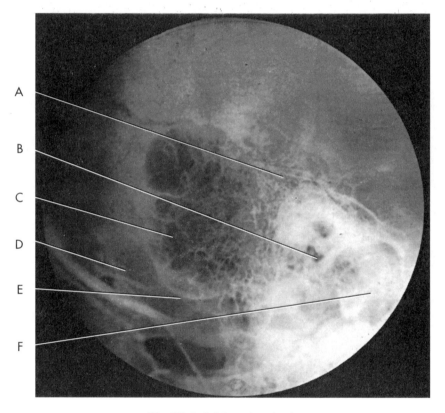

Fig. 23-1. Axiolateral projection.

Items 12 through 18 pertain to the axiolateral oblique projection (posterior profile; Stenvers method).

12. Where should a centering mark be located on the patient's face?

13. What three points of the face should be in contact with the x-ray table or vertical grid device?

14. The median sagittal plane should form an angle of _____ degrees with the plane of the film.

15. What positioning line of the head should be parallel with the transverse axis of the film?

16. How many degrees and in which direction should the central ray be directed?

17. What petrous pyramid is demonstrated in profile when the patient is facing toward the left shoulder? Is it the petrous pyramid closer to or farther from the film?

18. Identify each lettered structure in Figure 23-2.

A. _____   E. _____

B. _____   F. _____

C. _____   G. _____

D. _____

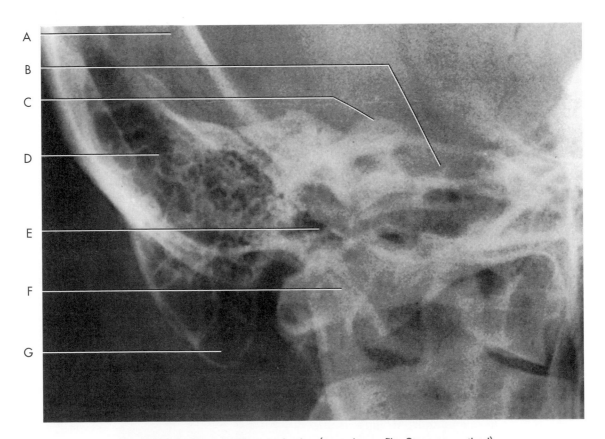

Fig. 23-2. Axiolateral oblique projection (posterior profile; Stenvers method).

Items 19 through 25 pertain to the axiolateral oblique projection (anterior profile; Arcelin method).

19. True or False. The median sagittal plane should be perpendicular to the film.

20. True or False. The infraorbitomeatal line should be perpendicular to the film.

21. True or False. A centering mark should be located approximately 1 inch (2.5 cm) anterior to the external acoustic (auditory) meatus.

22. What petrous pyramid is demonstrated in profile when the patient is facing toward the left shoulder? Is it the petrous pyramid closer to or farther from the film?

23. How many degrees and in which direction should the central ray be directed?

24. Where should the central ray enter the patient?

25. List the six evaluation criteria that indicate the patient was properly positioned for both the posterior profile projection (Stenvers method) and the anterior profile projection (Arcelin method).

Note to Students: Additional exercises referenced from Chapters 20, 21, 22, and 23 are found in the *Appendix: Supplemental Exercises for Skull Positioning* located in this workbook. Students should complete the review exercises for those chapters before completing the appendix exercises.

If your school has access to Mosby's Radiographic Instructional Series on Anatomy, Positioning, and Procedures, review Unit 23 at this time; your instructor may request that you respond to the series' exercises on paper. This unit covers the following essential projections:

Petromastoid portion
 Axiolateral (single tube-angulation; modified Law method)
 Axiolateral oblique (posterior profile; Stenvers method)
 Axiolateral oblique (anterior profile; Arcelin method)

Chapter 24
MAMMOGRAPHY

Part 1

ANATOMY AND PHYSIOLOGY OF THE BREAST

Instructions: Radiographers who perform mammography need to know the anatomy of the breast. This exercise pertains to the breast. Items require you to identify structures, fill in missing words, or provide a short answer.

1. Identify each lettered structure in Figure 24-1.

A. _____   C. _____

B. _____   D. _____

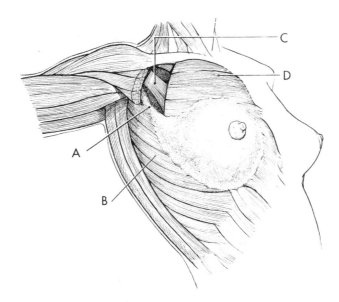

Fig. 24-1. Relationship of the breast to the chest wall.

2. Identify each lettered structure in Figure 24-2.

A. _____

B. _____

C. _____

D. _____

E. _____

F. _____

G. _____

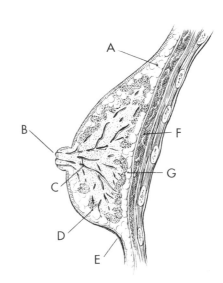

Fig. 24-2. Sagittal section through the female breast illustrating structural anatomy.

3. What is the function of the female breast?

4. Another term for the female breast is _____ gland.

5. The circular area of pigmented skin that surrounds the nipple is the _____.

6. The adult female breast contains _____ to _____ lobes.

7. The glandular elements found in the lobules of the female breast are the _____.

8. How does the patient's age affect the size of her breast lobules?

9. Define *involution*.

10. Normal involution replaces glandular and parenchymal tissues with increased amounts of _____.

11. What is the function of lactiferous ducts?

12. The axillary prolongation of the breast is also called the _____ of the breast.

13. The suspensory ligaments of the breast are called _____ ligaments.

14. Approximately 75% of the lymph drainage is toward the _____.

15. The internal mammary lymph nodes are situated behind the _____.

Part 2

RADIOGRAPHY OF THE BREAST

Instructions: Breast radiography, or mammography, is employed to demonstrate diseases of the breast. This exercise pertains to mammographic procedures. Items require you to fill in missing words or provide a short answer.

1. Name the two basic recording systems used for imaging the breast.

2. What mammographic recording system is the preferred method? Explain why.

3. What mammographic recording system is the most commonly used method?

4. Regardless of the system used for mammography, the entire examination should not produce a radiation dose to the patient that exceeds _____ rad.

5. What is the typical kilovoltage range used for film-screen mammography?

6. What is the typical kilovoltage used for xeromammography?

7. What material comprises the targets of standard x-ray tubes?

8. The material that comprises the targets of x-ray tubes used for film-screen mammography is _____.

9. The material that comprises the targets of x-ray tubes used for xeromammography is _____.

10. Why is tungsten not used for the target material of film-screen mammographic units?

11. Dedicated film-screen mammographic units use focal spots as small as _____ mm.

12. With reference to the patient, where should the cathode of the x-ray tube be positioned?

13. The source-to-image receptor distance (SID) for dedicated film-screen mammographic units should be at least _____ inches (_____ cm).

14. What is the purpose of compressing the breast for mammography?

15. Explain how breast compression affects exposure time.

16. Explain how breast compression affects radiographic density.

17. Explain how breast compression affects geometric distortion.

18. What is the major disadvantage of dedicated mammographic units?

19. Why should the breast be imaged without any cloth covering it?

20. Name the two standard projections routinely performed to demonstrate the breast.

21. Describe how the nipple should be positioned for both standard projections.

22. With reference to the breast, where should the side marker be placed on the film for the craniocaudal projection?

23. What standard projection requires the central ray to be angled other than vertically to the patient?

24. In what body position should the patient be placed for mammography?

25. How many exposures comprise the typical mammographic examination?

Self-Test: Mammography

Instructions: Answer the following questions by selecting the best choice.

1. The lymphatic vessels of the breast drain laterally into which lymph nodes?

   a. axillary
   b. thoracic
   c. abdominal
   d. internal mammary chain

2. The axillary prolongation of the breast is also called the _____ of the breast.

   a. tail
   b. body
   c. head
   d. wing

3. Which ducts function to drain milk from the lobes of the breast?

   a. axillary
   b. thoracic
   c. lymphatic
   d. lactiferous

4. How do breast tissues change after involution?

   a. Glandular tissues become dense and opaque.
   b. Parenchymal tissues become dense and opaque.
   c. Glandular tissues are replaced with fatty tissues.
   d. Fatty tissues are replaced with glandular tissues.

5. Which two projections comprise the standard examination to demonstrate the breasts?

   a. craniocaudal and lateromedial
   b. craniocaudal and mediolateral oblique
   c. caudocranial and lateromedial
   d. caudocranial and mediolateral oblique

6. Which projection requires the central ray to pass through the breast at an angle of 30 to 60 degrees?

   a. axillary
   b. caudocranial
   c. craniocaudal
   d. mediolateral oblique

7. Which muscle is often demonstrated with the craniocaudal projection?

   a. rectus abdominis
   b. pectoralis major
   c. serratus anterior
   d. lateral abdominal oblique

8. What is the purpose of compressing the breast for mammography?

   a. to reduce exposure time
   b. to decrease geometric distortion
   c. to produce uniform breast thickness
   d. to produce uniform radiographic density

9. Why is molybdenum rather than tungsten used for target material in dedicated film-screen mammography units?

   a. It has a higher tolerance for heat.
   b. It has a greater range of x-ray energies.
   c. It is more efficient in producing low-energy x-ray photons.
   d. It is more efficient in producing high-energy x-ray photons.

10. Why is film-screen mammography rather than xeromammography the preferred method for demonstrating the breast?

    a. It uses higher photon energies.
    b. It offers wider exposure latitude.
    c. It provides edge enhancement effect.
    d. It provides more detailed information.

If your school has access to Mosby's Radiographic Instructional Series on Anatomy, Positioning, and Procedures, review Unit 24 at this time; your instructor may request that you respond to the series' exercises on paper. This unit covers the following topics of special interest:

Risk versus benefit
Breast imaging
Method of examination
The augmented breast
Localization of nonpalpable lesions for biopsy
Breast specimen radiography
Examination of milk ducts

Chapter 25
CENTRAL NERVOUS SYSTEM

————— Part 1

ANATOMY OF THE
CENTRAL NERVOUS SYSTEM

Instructions: This exercise pertains to the anatomic structures of the central nervous system. Items require you to identify structures, fill in missing words, or provide a short answer.

1. Identify each lettered structure in Figure 25-1.

A. _____   E. _____

B. _____   F. _____

C. _____   G. _____

D. _____   H. _____

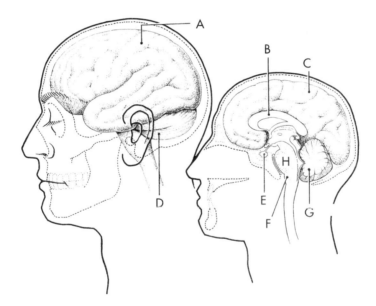

Fig. 25-1. Lateral surface and midsection of brain.

2. Identify each lettered structure in Figure 25-2.

A. _____

B. _____

C. _____

D. _____

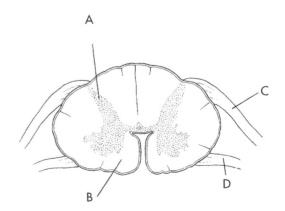

Fig. 25-2. Transverse section of spinal cord.

3. Identify each lettered structure in Figure 25-3.

A. _____

B. _____

C. _____

D. _____

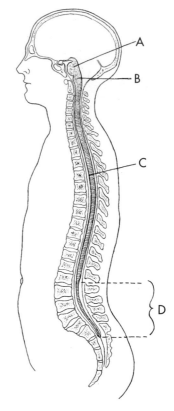

Fig. 25-3. Sagittal section showing spinal cord.

4. Identify each lettered structure in Figure 25-4.

A. _____   E. _____

B. _____   F. _____

C. _____   G. _____

D. _____   H. _____

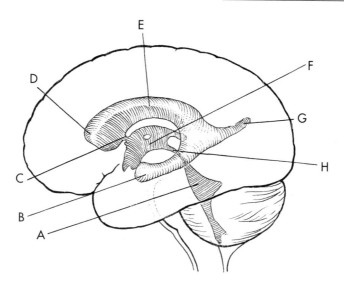

Fig. 25-4. Lateral aspect of cerebral ventricles in relation to surface of brain.

5. Identify each lettered structure in Figure 25-5.

A. _____

B. _____

C. _____

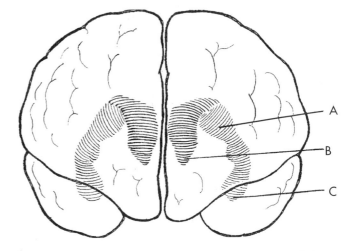

Fig. 25-5. Anterior aspect of lateral cerebral ventricles in relation to surface of brain.

6. Identify each lettered structure in Figure 25-6.

A. _____

B. _____

C. _____

D. _____

E. _____

F. _____

G. _____

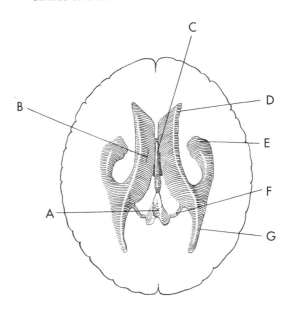

Fig. 25-6. Superior aspect of cerebral ventricles in relation to surface of brain.

7. Name the two main parts of the central nervous system.

8. Name the three parts of the brain.

9. Name the four parts of the brain stem.

10. Name the three parts of the hindbrain.

11. The largest part of the brain is the _____.

12. Another name for the cerebrum is the _____.

13. The stemlike portion of the brain that connects the cerebrum to the hindbrain is the _____.

14. The deep cleft that separates the cerebrum into right and left hemispheres is the _____

    _____.

15. Another name for the hypophysis cerebri is _____ _____.

16. The largest part of the hindbrain is the _____.

17. The portion of the hindbrain that connects the pons to the spinal cord is the _____ _____.

18. The protective membranes that enclose the brain and spinal cord are the _____.

19. The membrane that closely adheres to the brain and spinal cord is the _____ _____.

20. The outermost membrane that forms the tough fibrous covering for the brain and spinal cord is the

    _____ _____.

21. The two uppermost ventricles are called the right and left _____ ventricles.

22. The lateral ventricles are located in the portion of the brain called the _____.

23. Each lateral ventricle communicates with the third ventricle by way of the _____ foramen.

24. Another name for the interventricular foramen is _____ _____

    _____.

25. What are the two names for the passage between the third and fourth ventricles?

—————————— Part 2

RADIOGRAPHY OF THE CENTRAL NERVOUS SYSTEM

Instructions: This exercise pertains to examinations that demonstrate central nervous system structures. Items require you to provide a short answer.

1. Define *myelography.*

2. Identify three common sites for the injection of the contrast medium for myelography.

3. What abnormality is demonstrated with myelography?

4. What type or group of contrast media is preferred for myelography? Explain why.

5. When the exposure room is prepared for myelography, why should the spot-filming device be locked in place?

6. What should be done to reduce patient apprehension?

7. What are the two body positions most frequently used when the contrast medium is injected for myelography?

8. During myelography, what procedure controls the movement of the contrast medium after its injection?

9. During myelography, why should the patient hyperextend the neck?

10. When a traumatized patient with possible central nervous system involvement is radiographed, what should be the first radiograph made?

Self-Test: Central Nervous System

Instructions: Answer the following questions by selecting the best choice.

1. Which two structures comprise the central nervous system?

   a. brain and cerebellum
   b. brain and spinal cord
   c. cerebrum and cerebellum
   d. cerebrum and spinal cord

2. Which part of the brain is the forebrain?

   a. pons
   b. cerebrum
   c. cerebellum
   d. diencephalon

3. Which three parts of the central nervous system comprise the hindbrain?

   a. cerebrum, cerebellum, and spinal cord
   b. cerebrum, pons, and medulla oblongata
   c. pons, cerebellum, and medulla oblongata
   d. pons, spinal cord, and medulla oblongata

4. Which cerebral structure is the largest part of the brain?

   a. pons
   b. cerebrum
   c. cerebellum
   d. medulla oblongata

5. Which structure is divided into right and left hemispheres by the longitudinal fissure?

   a. pons
   b. cerebrum
   c. cerebellum
   d. medulla oblongata

6. What other term refers to the hypophysis cerebri?

   a. corpus callosum
   b. pituitary gland
   c. conus medullaris
   d. medulla spinalis

7. Which membrane forms the tough fibrous outer covering for the meninges?

   a. arachnoid
   b. pia mater
   c. dura mater

8. Which vessel connects the lateral ventricles to the third ventricle?

   a. cerebral aqueduct
   b. foramen of Luschka
   c. foramen of Magendie
   d. interventricular foramen

9. In which part of the brain is the fourth ventricle found?

   a. forebrain
   b. midbrain
   c. hindbrain

10. Which projection should be the first radiograph made on a traumatized patient with possible central nervous system involvement?

    a. AP axial
    b. AP oblique
    c. upright lateral
    d. cross-table lateral

11. Which examination is performed to demonstrate the contour of the subarachnoid space?

    a. myelography
    b. diskography
    c. pneumonography
    d. ventriculography

12. Which examination directly injects the contrast medium into fibrous cartilage between two vertebral bodies?

    a. myelography
    b. diskography
    c. pneumonography
    d. ventriculography

13. Which examination can evaluate the dynamic flow pattern of cerebral spinal fluid?

    a. myelography
    b. diskography
    c. pneumonography
    d. ventriculography

14. During myelography, which procedure should be performed to prevent contrast medium from entering the cerebral ventricles?

    a. Tilt the head of the table down.
    b. Have the patient hyperflex the neck.
    c. Have the patient hyperextend the neck.
    d. Position the patient lateral recumbent.

15. What is the purpose of tilting the table during myelography?

   a. to facilitate patient comfort
   b. to attach the footboard
   c. to control the flow of contrast medium
   d. to remove cerebral spinal fluid from the patient

If your school has access to Mosby's Radiographic Instructional Series on Anatomy, Positioning, and Procedures, review Unit 25 at this time; your instructor may request that you respond to the series' exercises on paper. This unit covers the following examinations:

Plain radiographic examination
Myelography
   Contrast media
   Computed tomography
Diskography
Chemonucleolysis
Magnetic resonance imaging
Cerebral pneumonography/ventriculography
Stereotactic surgery

Chapter 26
CIRCULATORY SYSTEM

Part 1

ANATOMY OF THE CIRCULATORY SYSTEM

Exercise 1

Instructions: This exercise pertains to the anatomy of the circulatory system. Items require you to identify structures.

1. Identify each lettered structure in Figure 26-1.

A. _____

B. _____

C. _____

D. _____

E. _____

F. _____

G. _____

H. _____

I. _____

J. _____

K. _____

L. _____

M. _____

N. _____

O. _____

P. _____

Q. _____

R. _____

S. _____

T. _____

U. _____

V. _____

W. _____

X. _____

Y. _____

Z. _____

AA. _____

BB. _____

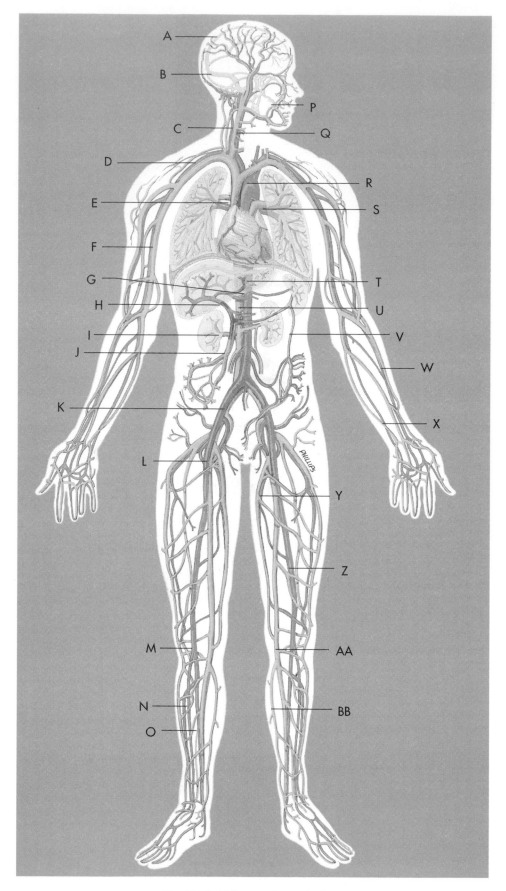

Fig. 26-1. Major arteries and veins.

2. Identify each lettered structure in Figure 26-2.

A. _____   H. _____

B. _____   I. _____

C. _____   J. _____

D. _____   K. _____

E. _____   L. _____

F. _____   M. _____

G. _____

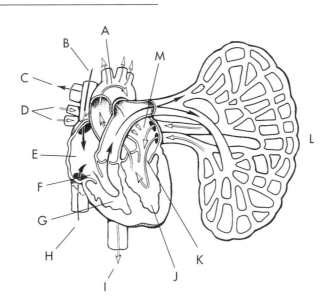

Fig. 26-2. The heart and great vessels. Black arrows indicate deoxygenated blood flow. White arrows indicate oxygenated blood flow.

3. Identify each lettered structure in Figure 26-3.

A. _____

B. _____

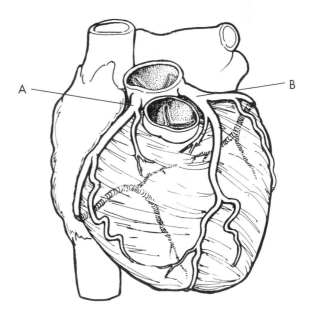

Fig. 26-3. Anterior view of coronary arteries.

4. Identify each lettered structure in Figure 26-4.

A. _____

B. _____

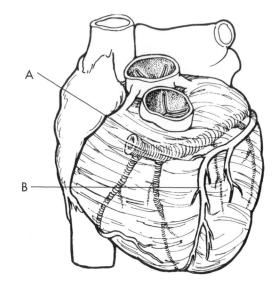

Fig. 26-4. Anterior view of coronary veins.

5. Identify each lettered structure in Figure 26-5.

A. _____

B. _____

C. _____

D. _____

E. _____

F. _____

G. _____

H. _____

I. _____

J. _____

K. _____

L. _____

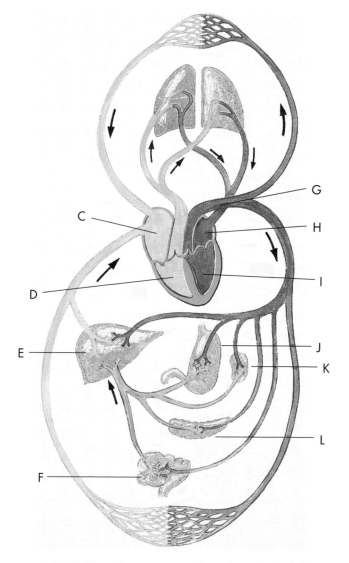

Fig. 26-5. The pulmonary, systemic, and portal circulation.

6. Identify each lettered structure in Figure 26-6.

A. _____

B. _____

C. _____

D. _____

E. _____

F. _____

G. _____

H. _____

I. _____

J. _____

K. _____

L. _____

M. _____

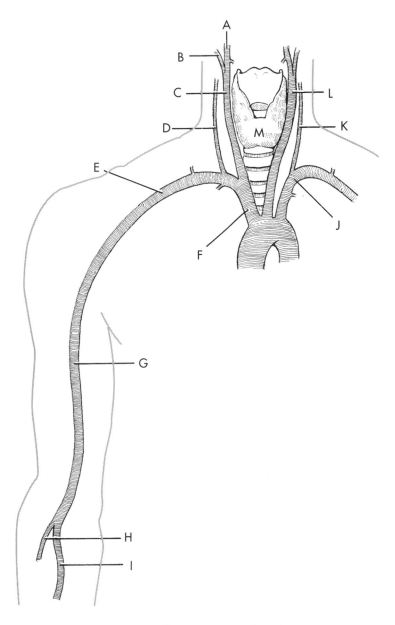

Fig. 26-6. Major arteries of upper chest, neck, and arm.

7. Identify each lettered structure in Figure 26-7.

A. _____   E. _____

B. _____   F. _____

C. _____   G. _____

D. _____

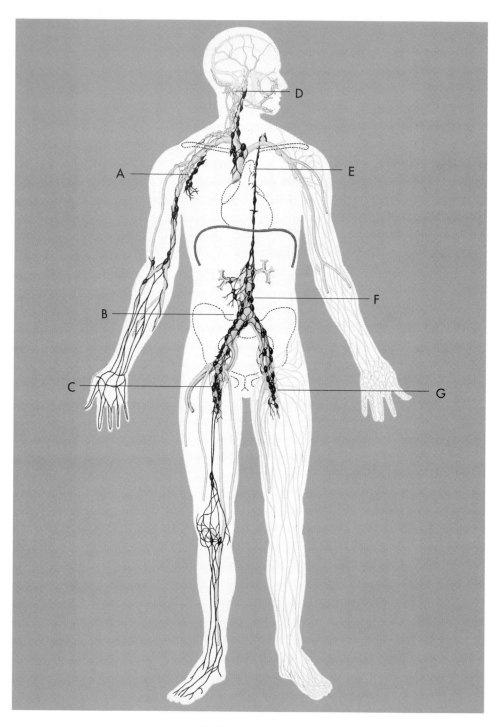

Fig. 26-7. Lymphatic system.

Exercise 2

Instructions: This exercise is a comprehensive review of the circulatory system. Items require you to fill in missing words or provide a short answer.

1. The circulatory system comprises two systems of related

   vessels, the _____ system and the

   _____ system.

2. The two systems that comprise the blood-vascular system

   are the _____ circulation and the

   _____ circulation.

3. The system that traverses the lungs to discharge carbon

   dioxide and take up oxygen is the _____
   circulation.

4. The vessels that convey blood away from the heart are

   collectively called _____.

5. The vessels that convey blood back toward the heart are

   collectively called _____.

6. Arteries subdivide to form _____.

7. Arterioles subdivide to form _____.

8. Capillaries unite to form _____.

9. The beginning branches for veins are _____.

10. Blood is transported to the left atrium by _____
    veins.

11. The major vein that returns blood from the upper parts of

    the body to the heart is the _____

    _____ _____.

12. The major vein that returns blood from the lower parts of

    the body to the heart is the _____

    _____ _____.

13. The muscular wall of the heart is the _____.

14. The membrane that lines the chambers of the heart is the

    _____.

15. The membrane that covers the heart is the _____.

16. Where in the heart is the myocardium the thickest? Explain why.

17. Where is the pericardial cavity?

18. The two upper chambers of the heart are the

    _____.

19. The two lower chambers of the heart are the

    _____.

20. The receiving chambers of the heart are the

    _____.

21. The distributing chambers of the heart are the

    _____.

22. Another name for the right atrioventricular valve is the

    _____ valve.

23. List two other terms that refer to the left atrioventricular valve.

24. What side of the heart handles venous (deoxygenated) blood?

25. What side of the heart handles arterial (oxygenated) blood?

26. What heart chamber pumps blood through the aortic valve?

27. The vessels that supply blood to the myocardium are the right and left _____ arteries.

28. The coronary sinus receives blood from the _____ veins.

29. The coronary sinus empties blood into the _____ atrium.

30. The great vessel that arises from the left ventricle to transport blood to the body is the _____.

31. The abdominal aorta divides into the right and left common _____ arteries.

32. The external iliac artery enters the lower limb and becomes the _____ artery.

33. The femoral artery passes blood into the _____ artery.

34. The popliteal artery bifurcates into the anterior and posterior _____ arteries.

35. The vessel that drains blood into the liver is the _____ vein.

36. The vessels that drain blood from the liver are the _____ veins.

37. Hepatic veins transport blood to the _____ _____ _____.

38. The large vessel that arises from the right atrium is the _____ artery.

39. The only arteries of the body that transport deoxygenated blood are the _____ arteries.

40. The only veins of the body that transport oxygenated blood are the _____ veins.

41. The contraction phase of the heart is called _____.

42. The relaxation phase of the heart is called _____.

43. List the four arteries that supply the brain.

44. Of the four trunk arteries that supply the brain, which one arises directly from the arch of the aorta?

45. The right and left vertebral arteries arise from the _____ arteries.

46. The right and left vertebral arteries unite to form the _____ artery.

47. Each common carotid artery bifurcates into _____ and _____ carotid arteries.

48. Each internal carotid artery bifurcates into anterior and middle _____ arteries.

49. The basilar artery bifurcates into the right and left _____ _____ arteries.

50. Blood is drained from the head by the _____ veins.

51. To reach the right subclavian artery, blood passes from the aorta through the _____ artery.

52. Blood passes from the brachiocephalic artery to the right _____ artery.

53. A subclavian artery supplies blood to the axillary artery

    and then to the _____ artery.

54. The brachial arteries bifurcate into the _____

    and _____ arteries.

55. The part of the body in which the cephalic vein originates

    is the _____.

56. The renal arteries arise from the _____.

57. The circle of Willis is located within the _____.

58. The central organ of the blood-vascular system is the

    _____.

59. The main terminal trunk of the lymphatic system is the

    _____ _____.

60. The thoracic duct drains its contents at the junction of the

    left _____ vein and the internal

    _____ vein.

──────────── Part 2

RADIOGRAPHY OF THE CIRCULATORY SYSTEM

Instructions: This exercise pertains to various radiographic examinations for the circulatory system. Because many of those procedures are dependent upon the preferences of the performing radiologist, most items are general in content rather than emphasize a specific procedure that may not be universally performed. Items require you to identify structures, fill in missing words, or provide a short answer.

1. List four reasons that catheterization is preferred over direct injection of the contrast medium through a needle.

2. The most widely used method of catheterization is the _____ technique.

3. The preferred site for insertion of the catheter for most selective angiography is the _____ artery.

4. What is the purpose of side holes near the tip of the catheter?

5. List symptoms of a vasovagal reaction caused by the injection of the contrast medium.

6. What treatment should be given to the patient who is experiencing low blood pressure because of a vasovagal reaction?

7. List three symptoms of shock.

8. In preparation for angiography, why should the patient be prevented from consuming solid food?

9. In preparation for angiography, why should the patient be allowed to drink clear liquids?

10. For thoracic aortography, all projections should direct a perpendicular central ray to the level of the _____ vertebra.

11. Identify each lettered structure in Figure 26-8.

A. _____   E. _____

B. _____   F. _____

C. _____   G. _____

D. _____   H. _____

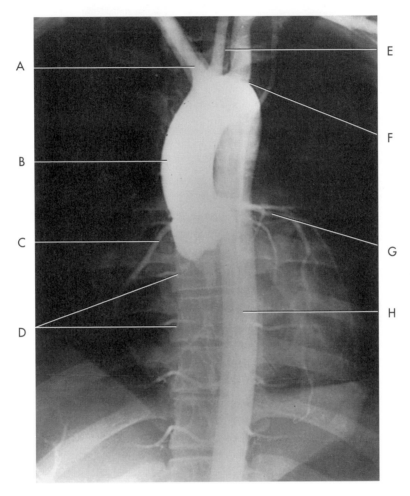

Fig. 26-8. AP thoracic aortogram.

12. How much of the aorta should be imaged for abdominal aortography?

13. For abdominal aortography, which projection of the abdominal aorta—AP or lateral—best demonstrates the celiac and superior mesenteric artery origins?

14. Identify each lettered structure in Figure 26-9.

A. _____   D. _____

B. _____   E. _____

C. _____   F. _____

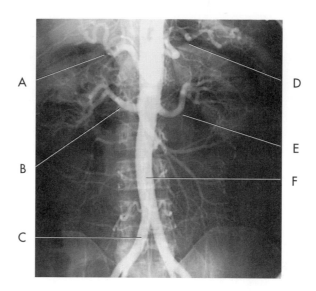

Fig. 26-9. AP abdominal aortogram.

15. Identify each lettered structure in Figure 26-10.

A. _____   C. _____

B. _____

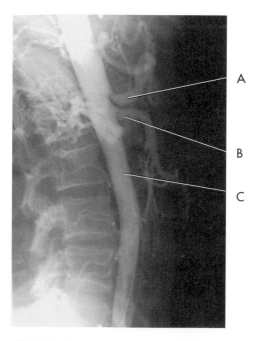

Fig. 26-10. Lateral abdominal aortogram.

16. For pulmonary arteriography, which projection—AP or lateral—should use a compensating (trough) filter to obtain a radiograph with more uniform density between the vertebrae and the lungs?

17. All radiographs for selective abdominal visceral arteriography should be exposed during suspended _____ (inspiration or expiration).

18. Identify each lettered structure in Figure 26-11.

A. _____   D. _____

B. _____   E. _____

C. _____

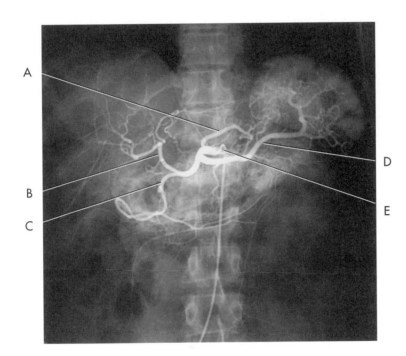

Fig. 26-11. Selective AP celiac arteriogram.

19. Why is it advantageous to examine the patient's intravenous urography radiographs before positioning the patient for a renal arteriogram?

20. For demonstrating the portal venous system, the contrast medium should be injected into the _____ artery.

21. Blood in veins flows _____ (proximally or distally).

22. For renal venography, the renal vein is most easily catheterized from the _____ (upper or lower) limb approach.

23. To best demonstrate the superior vena cava, the catheter should be positioned into the _____ vein.

24. To best demonstrate the inferior vena cava, the catheter should be positioned into a _____

    _____ vein.

25. The arteries of an entire upper limb can be opacified with a single injection of contrast medium if the catheter is positioned

    into the _____ artery.

26. Identify each lettered structure in Figure 26-12.

A. _____   C. _____

B. _____   D. _____

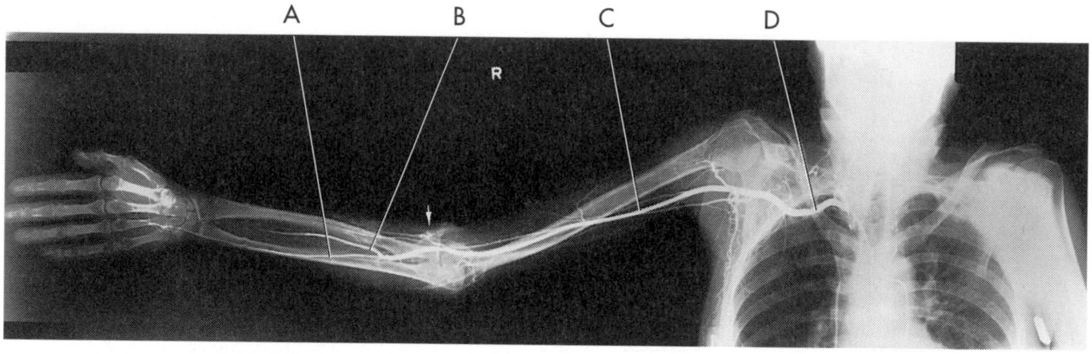

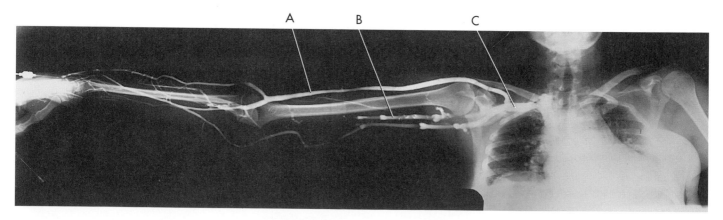

Fig. 26-12. Right upper limb arteriogram (radial artery not demonstrated due to occlusion).

27. Where is the injection site for the introduction of contrast medium for upper limb venography?

28. Identify each lettered structure in Figure 26-13.

A. _____   C. _____

B. _____

Fig. 26-13. Right upper limb venogram.

29. For simultaneous bilateral femoral arteriograms, how should the patient's legs be positioned?

30. Identify each lettered structure in Figure 26-14.

A. _____

B. _____

C. _____

D. _____

E. _____

F. _____

G. _____

H. _____

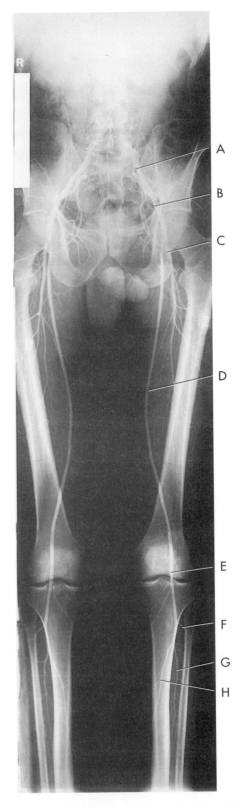

Fig. 26-14. Normal aortofemoral arteriogram in late arterial phase.

31. At what area of the leg should radiographs begin for lower limb venography?

32. For lower limb venography, what is the purpose of applying tourniquets just proximal to the ankle and knee?

33. For cerebral angiography, approximately how many seconds does it take for blood to flow from the internal carotid artery to the jugular vein?

34. For cerebral arteriography, why should the first radiograph of the series be made before the arrival of the contrast medium?

35. List the three phases of blood flow that should be seen in cerebral angiography.

36. Figures 26-15, 26-16, and 26-17 are cerebral angiograms, each showing a phase of blood flow. Examine each image and identify the phase of blood flow the image represents.

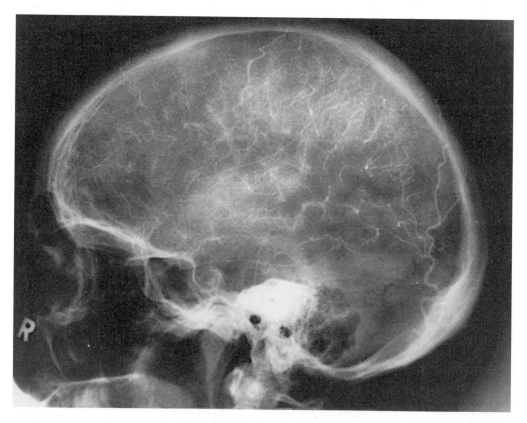

Fig. 26-15. Cerebral angiogram.

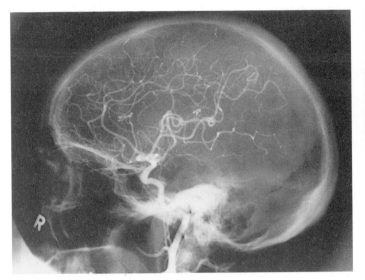

Fig. 26-16. Cerebral angiogram.

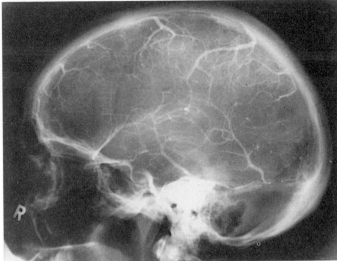

Fig. 26-17. Cerebral angiogram.

a. Figure 26-15: _____

b. Figure 26-16: _____

c. Figure 26-17: _____

37. For the basic AP projection during cerebral angiography, what positioning line of the skull should be perpendicular to the horizontal plane?

38. For the AP axial projection (supraorbital) to demonstrate anterior circulation during cerebral angiography, how should the central ray be directed to project the vessels above the floor of the anterior cranial fossa?

39. For the AP axial oblique projection (transorbital) to demonstrate anterior circulation during cerebral angiography, in which direction (toward the injected side or away from the injected side) should the head be rotated?

40. For the AP axial oblique projection (transorbital) to demonstrate the internal carotid bifurcation and the anterior communicating and middle cerebral arteries within the orbital shadow, how should the central ray be directed?

Self-Test: Anatomy and Radiography of the Circulatory System

Instructions: Answer the following questions by selecting the best choice.

1. Which vessels originate immediately because of the division of arteries?

   a. veins
   b. venules
   c. arterioles
   d. capillaries

2. In which portion of the body is the basilic vein located?

   a. head
   b. abdomen
   c. lower limb
   d. upper limb

3. Which chamber of the heart receives deoxygenated blood?

   a. left atrium
   b. left ventricle
   c. right atrium
   d. right ventricle

4. Which chamber of the heart receives pulmonary veins?

   a. left atrium
   b. left ventricle
   c. right atrium
   d. right ventricle

5. What is the purpose of the septa of the heart?

   a. to separate atria from ventricles
   b. to provide openings into the atria
   c. to form the atrioventricular valves
   d. to divide the heart into right and left halves

6. The circuit for blood flow from the left ventricle to the right atrium is the _____ circulation.

   a. deep
   b. systemic
   c. pulmonary
   d. superficial

7. Which arteries are the first to branch from the ascending aorta?

   a. coronary
   b. vertebral
   c. subclavian
   d. common carotid

8. Through which valve does blood pass when it exits the heart for systemic circulation?

   a. mitral
   b. aortic
   c. bicuspid
   d. tricuspid

9. A disadvantage of nonionic contrast agents when compared with ionic contrast agents of lower iodine concentrations is:

   a. increased viscosity.
   b. increased cardiovascular side effects.
   c. increased exposure factor requirements.
   d. decreased radiographic contrast of opacified vessels.

10. Why are exposures in both planes unable to occur at the same moment during simultaneous biplane imaging?

   a. X-ray tubes will overload.
   b. Scatter radiation will fog the films.
   c. Two injections of contrast medium are required.
   d. X-ray generators cannot be synchronized for multiple exposures.

11. Which procedure should be performed to reduce magnification of structures for the lateral projection during thoracic aortography?

   a. Increase the source-to-image receptor distance (SID).
   b. Increase the object-to-image receptor distance (OID).
   c. Use a cassette changer.
   d. Use the smallest available focal spot.

12. Which arteriogram requires the use of a compensating (trough) filter to obtain a more uniform density between vertebral structures and lungs?

   a. AP pulmonary
   b. AP celiac axis
   c. lateral pulmonary
   d. AP superior mesenteric

13. To which level of the patient should the film and central ray be centered for the AP abdominal aortogram?

   a. T6
   b. T10
   c. L2
   d. iliac crests

14. To which level of the patient should the film and central ray be centered for the celiac arteriogram?

   a. T2
   b. T6
   c. L2
   d. S1

15. Which area of the patient should be prepared for the contrast medium injection for cephalic venography?

   a. thigh
   b. ankle
   c. wrist
   d. upper arm

16. Which area of the patient should be prepared for the contrast medium injection to demonstrate the superior vena cava?

   a. thigh
   b. ankle
   c. wrist
   d. upper arm

17. Which area of the patient is the preferred site for insertion of the catheter through the skin for internal carotid arteriography?

   a. neck
   b. thigh
   c. abdomen
   d. upper arm

18. Why should a radiograph be taken before the arrival of contrast medium for cerebral angiography?

   a. to serve as a subtraction mask
   b. to ensure that collimation is adequate
   c. to check for proper patient positioning
   d. to verify that correct exposure factors are used

19. Which phase of blood flow should have the most films exposed during cerebral angiography?

   a. venous
   b. arterial
   c. capillary
   d. parenchymal

20. Which positioning line of the skull should be perpendicular to the horizontal plane for basic AP projections during cerebral arteriography?

   a. orbitomeatal
   b. acanthomeatal
   c. glabellomeatal
   d. infraorbitomeatal

If your school has access to Mosby's Radiographic Instructional Series on Anatomy, Positioning, and Procedures, review Unit 26 at this time; your instructor may request that you respond to the series' exercises on paper. This unit covers selected aspects of the following examinations:

Diagnostic visceral and peripheral angiography
Cerebral angiography
Interventional radiology
Lymphography
Photographic subtraction technique

Chapter 27
SECTIONAL ANATOMY FOR RADIOGRAPHERS

Chapter 27 Review

Instructions: An understanding by the radiographer of the relationships between organ and skeletal structures is essential in computed tomography, magnetic resonance imaging, and diagnostic ultrasound examinations because all three modalities create images of sectional anatomy. This exercise is a review of sectional anatomy. Items require you to identify structures.

Figure 27-1 is a CT localizer, or scout, image of the skull. Figures 27-2 through 27-5 pertain to the imaging planes shown in Figure 27-1.

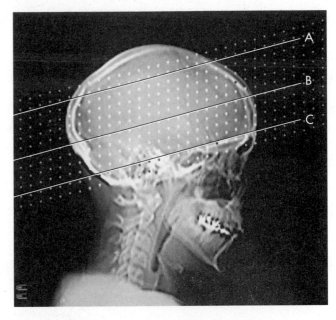

Fig. 27-1. CT localizer, or scout, image of the skull.

1. Identify each lettered structure in Figure 27-2.

A. _____

B. _____

C. _____

D. _____

E. _____

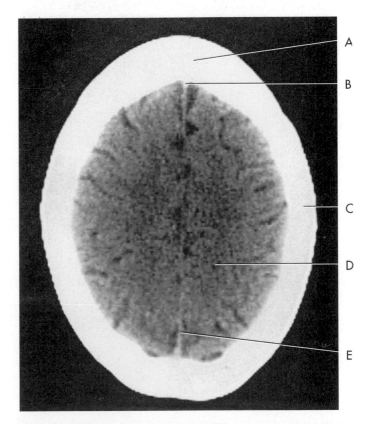

Fig. 27-2. Computed tomography (CT) image corresponding to level A in Fig. 27-1.

2. Identify each lettered structure in Figure 27-3.

A. _____   F. _____

B. _____   G. _____

C. _____   H. _____

D. _____   I. _____

E. _____   J. _____

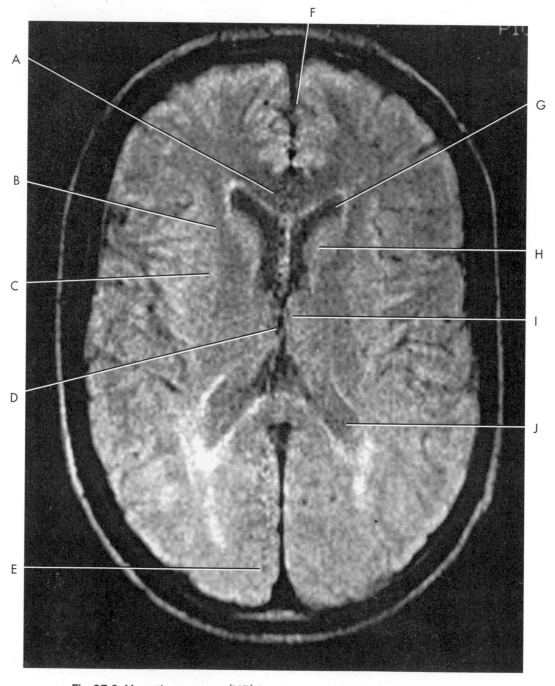

Fig. 27-3. Magnetic resonance (MR) image corresponding to level B in Fig. 27-1.

3. Identify each lettered structure in Figure 27-4.

A. _____   G. _____

B. _____   H. _____

C. _____   I. _____

D. _____   J. _____

E. _____   K. _____

F. _____

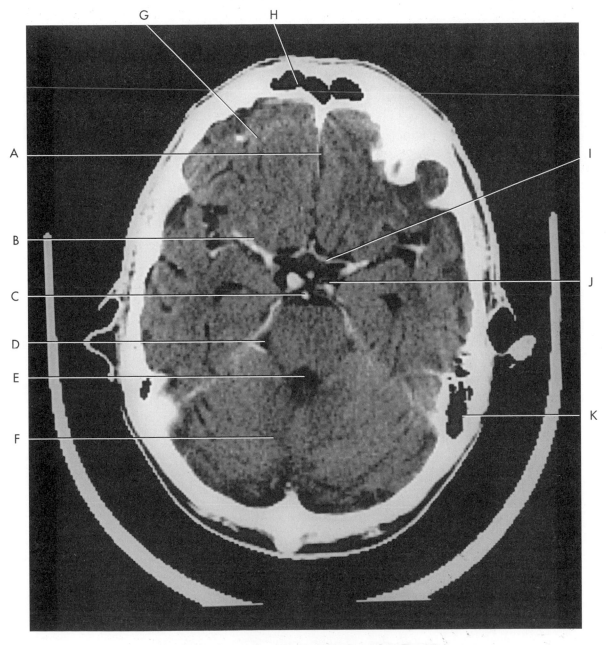

Fig. 27-4. CT image corresponding to level C in Fig. 27-1.

4. Identify each lettered structure in Figure 27-5.

A. _____   G. _____

B. _____   H. _____

C. _____   I. _____

D. _____   J. _____

E. _____   K. _____

F. _____

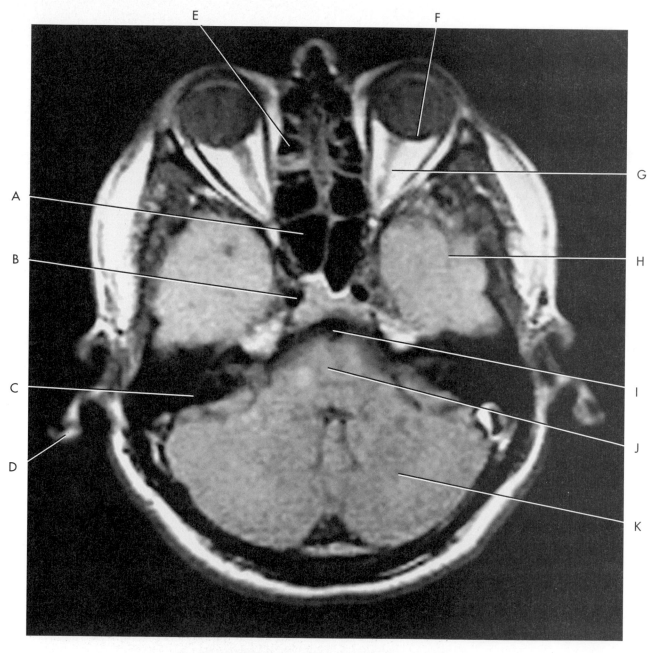

Fig. 27-5. MR image corresponding to level C in Fig. 27-1.

5. Identify each lettered structure in **Figure 27-6**.

A. _____

B. _____

C. _____

D. _____

E. _____

F. _____

G. _____

H. _____

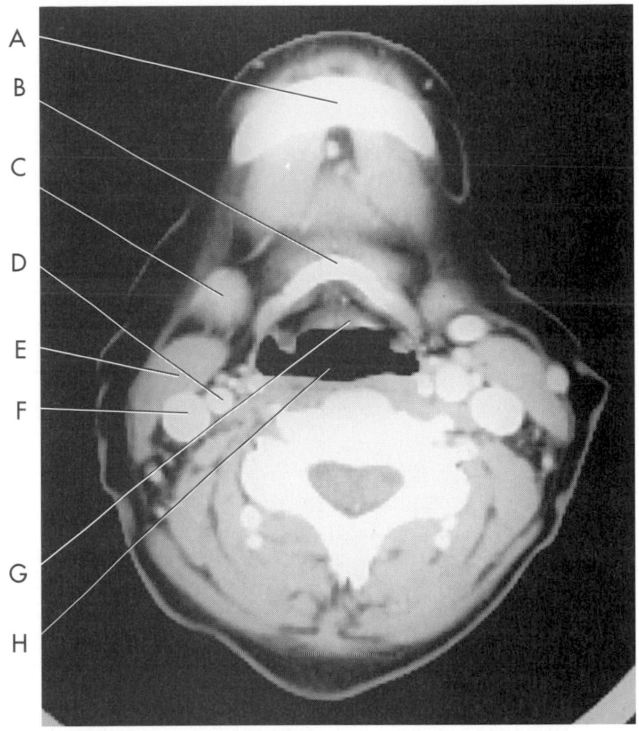

Fig. 27-6. CT image through the fourth cervical vertebra.

6. Identify each lettered structure in Figure 27-7.

A. _____

B. _____

C. _____

D. _____

E. _____

F. _____

G. _____

H. _____

I. _____

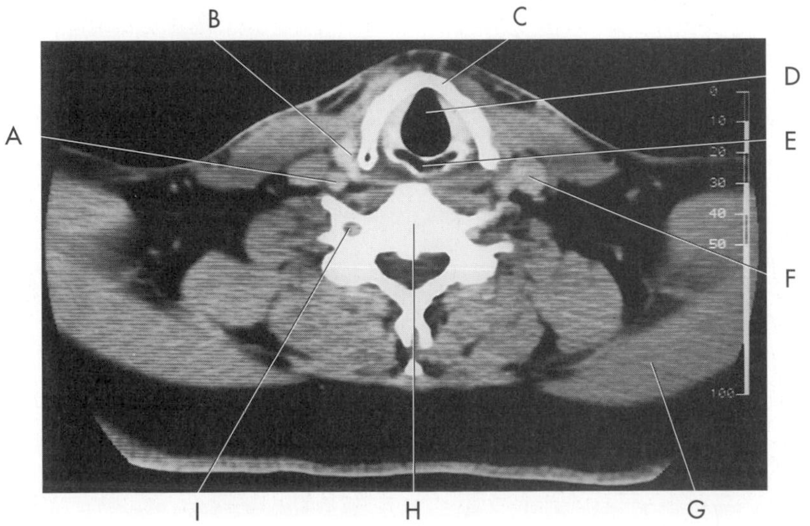

Fig. 27-7. CT image through the sixth cervical vertebra.

7. Identify each lettered structure in Figure 27-8.

A. _____

B. _____

C. _____

D. _____

E. _____

F. _____

G. _____

H. _____

I. _____

J. _____

K. _____

L. _____

M. _____

N. _____

O. _____

P. _____

Q. _____

R. _____

S. _____

T. _____

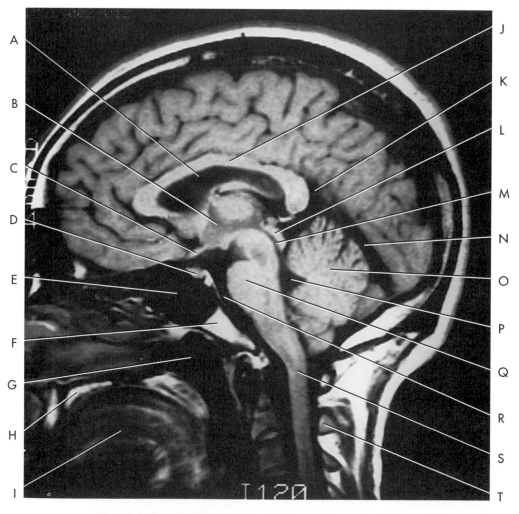

Fig. 27-8. Sagittal MR image through the median sagittal plane.

Figure 27-9 is a CT localizer, or scout, image of the skull. Figures 27-10, 27-11, and 27-12 pertain to the imaging planes shown in Figure 27-9.

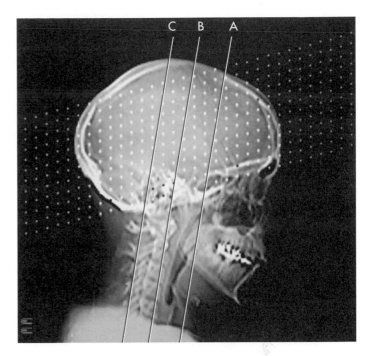

Fig. 27-9. CT localizer, or scout, image of the skull.

8. Identify each lettered structure in Figure 27-10.

A. _____

B. _____

C. _____

D. _____

E. _____

F. _____

G. _____

H. _____

I. _____

J. _____

K. _____

L. _____

M. _____

N. _____

O. _____

P. _____

Q. _____

R. _____

S. _____

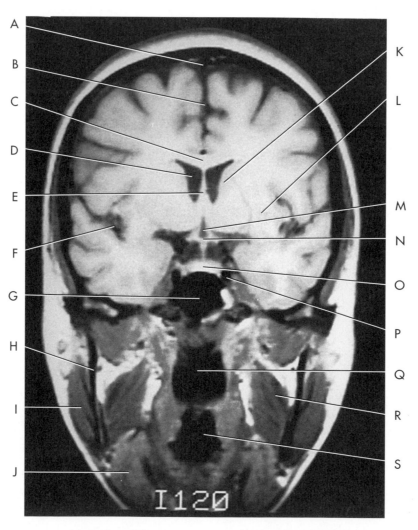

Fig. 27-10. Coronal MR image corresponding to level A in Fig. 27-9.

9. Identify each lettered structure in Figure 27-11.

A. _____   G. _____

B. _____   H. _____

C. _____   I. _____

D. _____   J. _____

E. _____   K. _____

F. _____

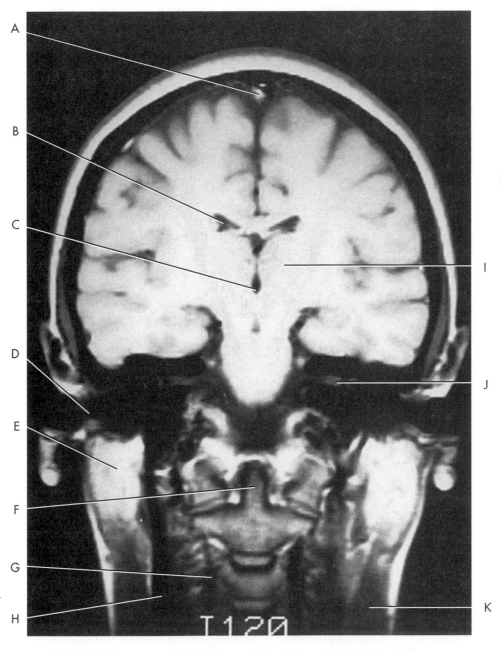

Fig. 27-11. Coronal MR image corresponding to level B in Fig. 27-9.

10. Identify each lettered structure in Figure 27-12.

A. _____

B. _____

C. _____

D. _____

E. _____

F. _____

G. _____

H. _____

I. _____

J. _____

K. _____

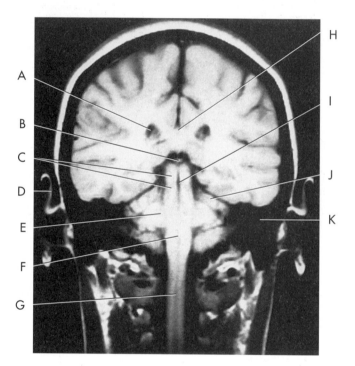

Fig. 27-12. Coronal MR image corresponding to level C in Fig. 27-9.

Figure 27-13 is a CT localizer, or scout, image of the thorax. Figures 27-14, 27-15, and 27-16 pertain to the imaging planes shown in Figure 27-13.

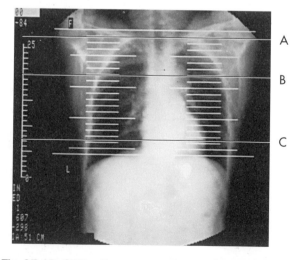

Fig. 27-13. CT localizer, or scout, image of the thorax.

11. Identify each lettered structure in Figure 27-14.

A. _____   F. _____

B. _____   G. _____

C. _____   H. _____

D. _____   I. _____

E. _____   J. _____

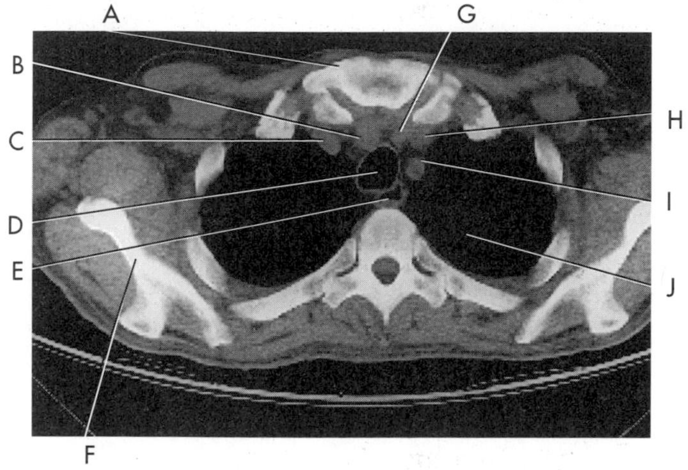

Fig. 27-14. CT image corresponding to level A at the second thoracic vertebra in Fig. 27-13.

12. Identify each lettered structure in Figure 27-15.

A. _____   G. _____

B. _____   H. _____

C. _____   I. _____

D. _____   J. _____

E. _____   K. _____

F. _____

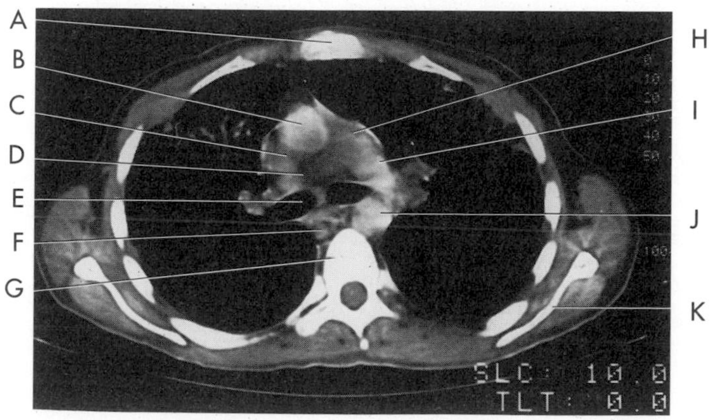

Fig. 27-15. CT image corresponding to level B at the fifth thoracic vertebra in Fig. 27-13.

13. Identify each lettered structure in Figure 27-16.

A. _____   G. _____

B. _____   H. _____

C. _____   I. _____

D. _____   J. _____

E. _____   K. _____

F. _____

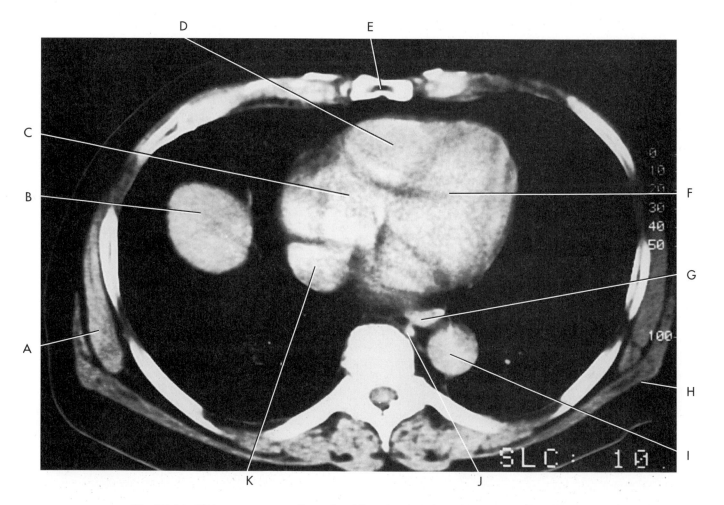

Fig. 27-16. CT image corresponding to level C at the ninth thoracic vertebra in Fig. 27-13.

14. Identify each lettered structure in Figure 27-17.

A. _____   G. _____

B. _____   H. _____

C. _____   I. _____

D. _____   J. _____

E. _____   K. _____

F. _____   L. _____

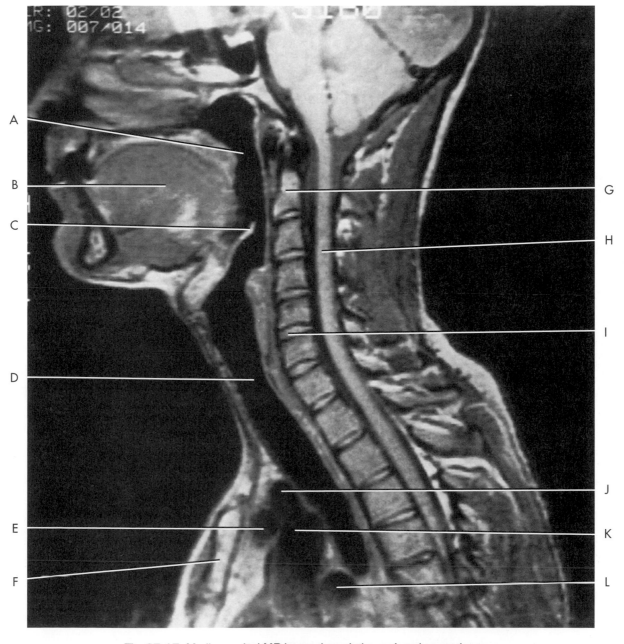

Fig. 27-17. Median sagittal MR image through the neck and upper thorax.

15. Identify each lettered structure in Figure 27-18.

A. _____

B. _____

C. _____

D. _____

E. _____

F. _____

G. _____

H. _____

I. _____

J. _____

K. _____

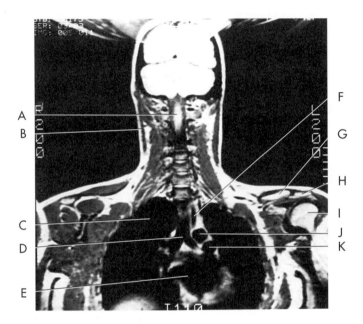

Fig. 27-18. MR image of the neck and thorax through the median coronal plane.

Figure 27-19 is a CT localizer, or scout, image of the abdominopelvic region. Figures 27-20 through 27-26 pertain to the imaging planes shown in Figure 27-19.

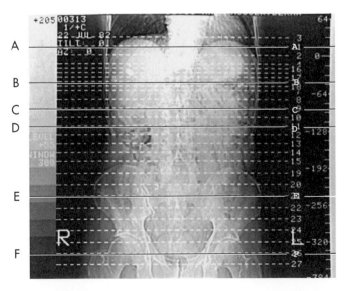

Fig. 27-19. CT localizer, or scout, image of the abdominopelvic region.

16. Identify each lettered structure in Figure 27-20.

A. _____

B. _____

C. _____

D. _____

E. _____

F. _____

G. _____

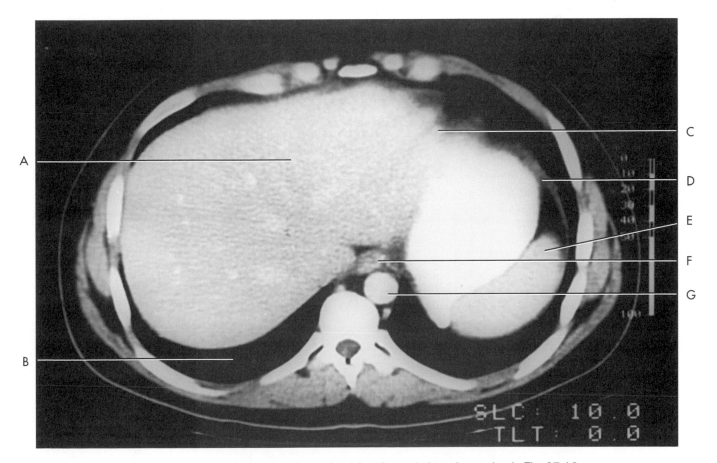

Fig. 27-20. CT image corresponding to level A at the tenth thoracic vertebra in Fig. 27-19.

17. Identify each lettered structure in Figure 27-21.

A. _____   G. _____

B. _____   H. _____

C. _____   I. _____

D. _____   J. _____

E. _____   K. _____

F. _____

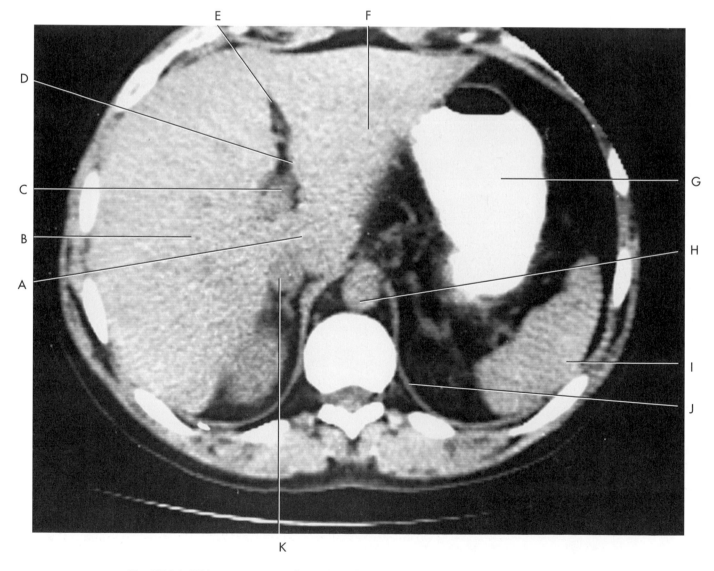

Fig. 27-21. CT image corresponding to level B at the twelfth thoracic vertebra in Fig. 27-19.

18. Identify each lettered structure in Figure 27-22.

A. _____

B. _____

C. _____

D. _____

E. _____

F. _____

G. _____

H. _____

I. _____

J. _____

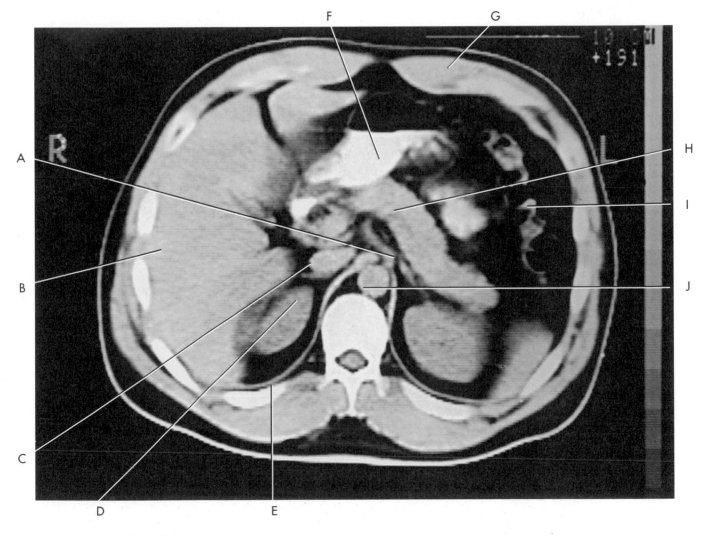

Fig. 27-22. CT image corresponding to level C at the second lumbar vertebra in Fig. 27-19.

19. Identify each lettered structure in Figure 27-23.

A. _____   E. _____

B. _____   F. _____

C. _____   G. _____

D. _____

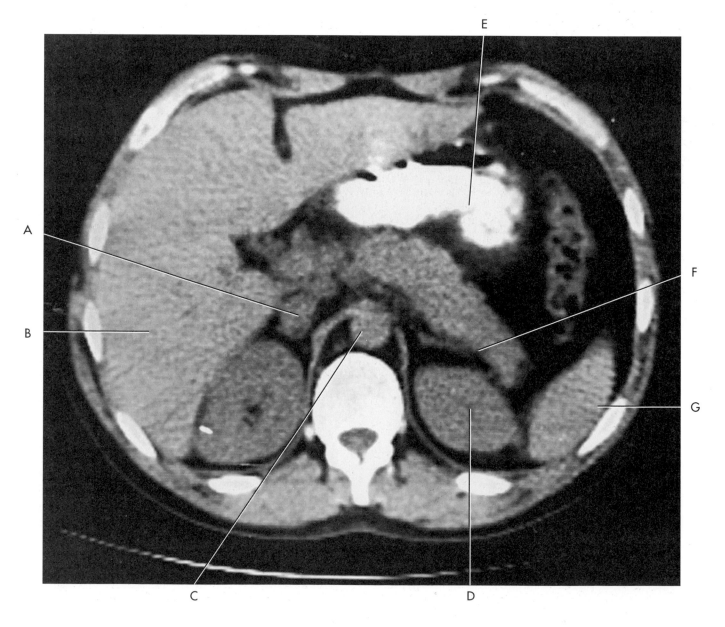

Fig. 27-23. CT image corresponding to level D at the interspace between the second and third lumbar vertebrae in Fig. 27-19.

20. Identify each lettered structure in Figure 27-24.

A. _____

B. _____

C. _____

D. _____

E. _____

F. _____

G. _____

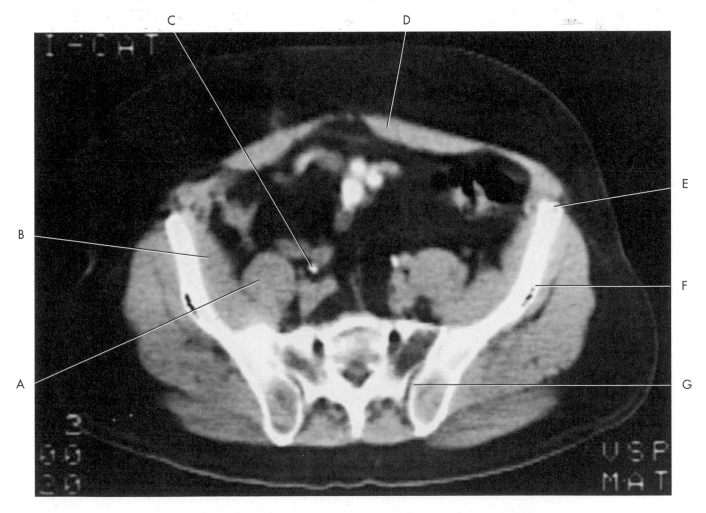

Fig. 27-24. CT image corresponding to level E at the anterior superior iliac spine (ASIS) in Fig. 27-19.

21. Identify each lettered structure in Figure 27-25.

A. _____   E. _____

B. _____   F. _____

C. _____   G. _____

D. _____

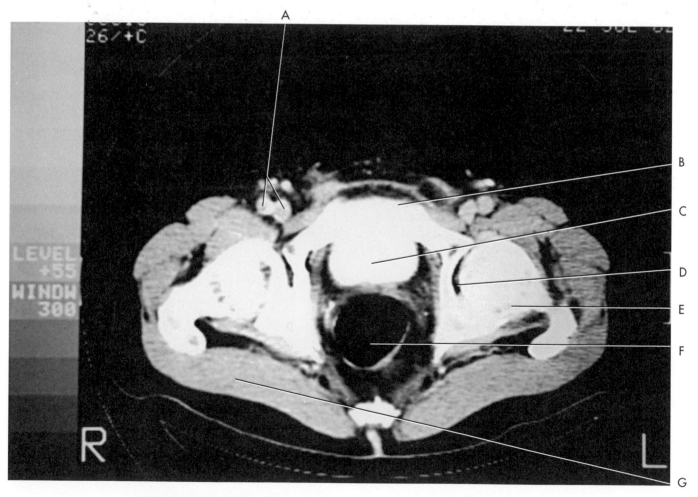

Fig. 27-25. CT image corresponding to level F at the coccyx (female) in Fig. 27-19.

22. Identify each lettered structure in Figure 27-26.

A. _____

B. _____

C. _____

D. _____

E. _____

F. _____

G. _____

H. _____

I. _____

J. _____

K. _____

L. _____

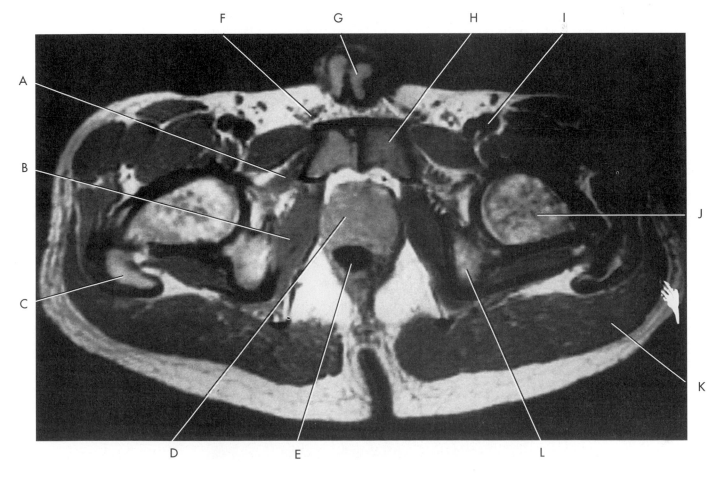

Fig. 27-26. CT image corresponding to level F at the coccyx (male) in Fig. 27-19.

23. Identify each lettered structure in Figure 27-27.

A. _____   H. _____

B. _____   I. _____

C. _____   J. _____

D. _____   K. _____

E. _____   L. _____

F. _____   M. _____

G. _____

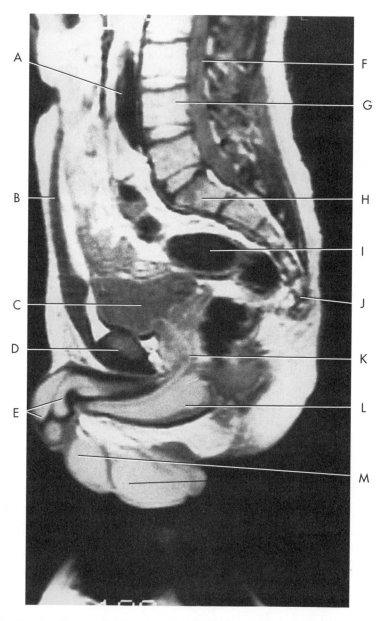

Fig. 27-27. MR image of the abdominopelvic region at the median sagittal plane.

24. Identify each lettered structure in Figure 27-28.

A. _____

B. _____

C. _____

D. _____

E. _____

F. _____

G. _____

H. _____

I. _____

J. _____

K. _____

L. _____

M. _____

N. _____

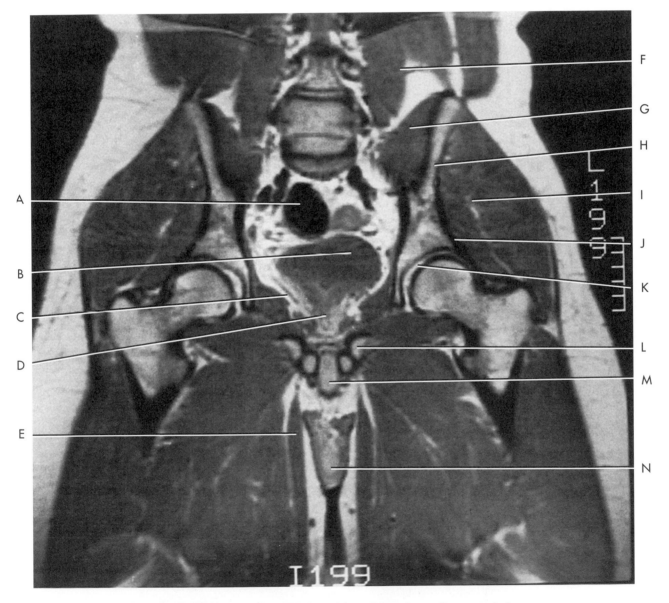

Fig. 27-28. MR image of the abdominopelvic region at the median coronal plane.

If your school has access to Mosby's Radiographic Instructional Series on Anatomy, Positioning, and Procedures, review Unit 27 at this time; your instructor may request that you respond to the series' exercises on paper. This unit covers the examination techniques for the following anatomic regions:

Cranial region
Thoracic region
Abdominopelvic region

Appendix

SUPPLEMENTAL EXERCISES FOR SKULL POSITIONING

Note to Students: The exercises and self-test in this appendix pertain to information referenced from Chapters 20, 21, 22, and 23. They should be completed after the review exercises for those four chapters have been completed.

Skull Positioning Review

Exercise 1

Instructions: Match each projection in Column A with the number of degrees and direction of central ray angulation in Column B. Not all central ray angulations may apply to the listed projections, and some angulations may be used more than once.

Column A

____ 1. AP axial (TMJ)

____ 2. AP axial (facial bones)

____ 3. AP axial (cranium; Towne method)

____ 4. PA (sphenoidal sinuses)

____ 5. PA axial (cranium; Caldwell method)

____ 6. PA axial (cranium; Haas method)

____ 7. PA axial (sinuses; original Caldwell method)

____ 8. axiolateral oblique (TMJ)

____ 9. axiolateral oblique (mandible; patient upright)

____ 10. axiolateral oblique (mandible; patient semisupine)

____ 11. axiolateral oblique (anterior profile; Arcelin method)

____ 12. axiolateral oblique (posterior profile; Stenvers method)

____ 13. parietoacanthial (sinuses; Waters method)

____ 14. parieto-orbital oblique (optic foramen; Rhese method)

____ 15. axiolateral (mastoids; single tube-angulation method [Law method])

Column B

a. perpendicular

b. 10 degrees caudad

c. 10 degrees cephalad

d. 12 degrees caudad

e. 12 degrees cephalad

f. 15 degrees caudad

g. 15 degrees cephalad

h. 20 degrees caudad

i. 20 degrees cephalad

j. 23 degrees caudad

k. 23 degrees cephalad

l. 25 degrees caudad

m. 25 degrees cephalad

n. 30 degrees caudad

o. 30 degrees cephalad

p. 35 degrees caudad

q. 35 degrees cephalad

r. 37 degrees cephalad

Exercise 2

Instructions: Match the projections in Column A with the locations in Column B. Each location in Column B is either a centering point for the body part or a point where the central ray should enter or exit the patient. Not all locations may apply to the listed projections.

Column A

_____ 1. AP axial (TMJ)

_____ 2. AP axial (zygomatic arches)

_____ 3. lateral (cranium)

_____ 4. lateral (nasal bones)

_____ 5. lateral (facial bones)

_____ 6. lateral (sella turcica)

_____ 7. lateral (paranasal sinuses)

_____ 8. PA (mandibular rami)

_____ 9. PA axial (cranium; Caldwell method)

_____ 10. PA axial (cranium; Haas method)

_____ 11. parietoacanthial (Waters method)

_____ 12. axiolateral oblique (TMJ)

_____ 13. axiolateral oblique (mandible)

_____ 14. axiolateral oblique (posterior profile; Stenvers method)

_____ 15. axiolateral (mastoids; single tube-angulation method [Law method])

Column B

a. nasion

b. glabella

c. acanthion

d. zygomatic bone

e. 3/4 inch (1.9 cm) distal to the nasion

f. 11/2 inches (3.7 cm) above the nasion

g. 3 inches (7.5 cm) above the nasion

h. slightly posterior to the gonion

i. external acoustic (auditory) meatus

j. 1/2 inch (1.2 cm) anterior to the external acoustic meatus

k. 1 inch (2.5 cm) anterior to the external acoustic meatus

l. 1 inch (2.5 cm) posterior to the external acoustic meatus

m. 3/4 inch (1.9 cm) anterior and 3/4 inch (1.9 cm) superior to the external acoustic meatus

n. 2 inches (5 cm) superior to the external acoustic meatus

o. tip of the nose to the midpoint of the film

p. 1/2 to 1 inch (1.2 to 2.5 cm) posterior to the outer canthus

Exercise 3

Instructions: Figure A shows diagrams of various projections of the skull (cranium, facial bones, sinuses, etc.). Listed below the diagrams are names and characteristics of projections of the skull. Identify in the space provided the diagram that applies to each name or characteristic. Not all diagrams may apply, and some diagrams may be used more than once.

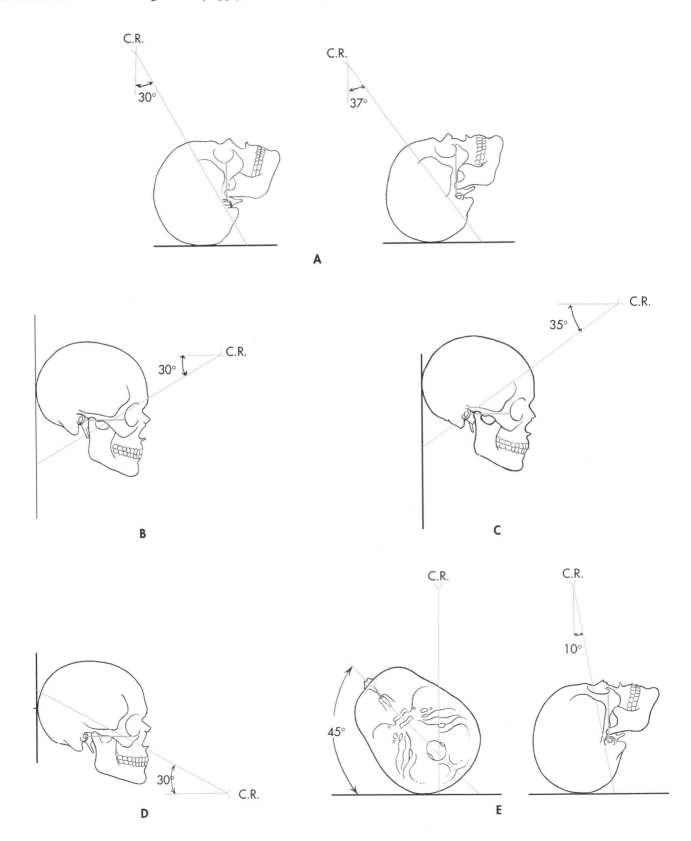

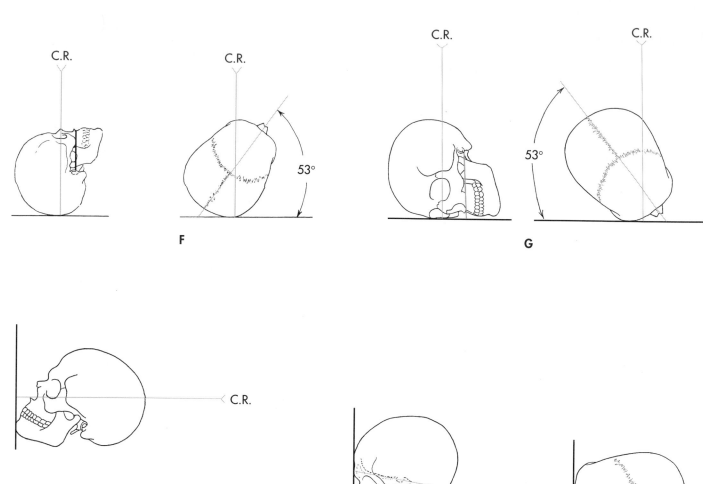

F

G

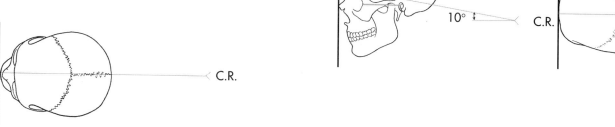

H

I

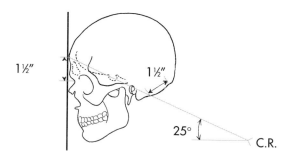

J

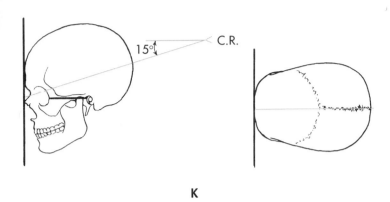

K

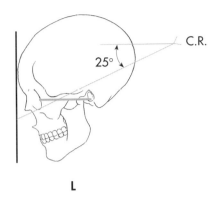

L

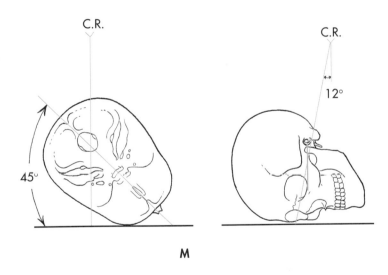

M

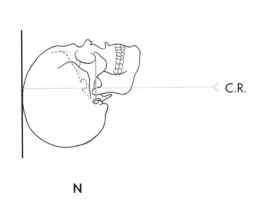

N

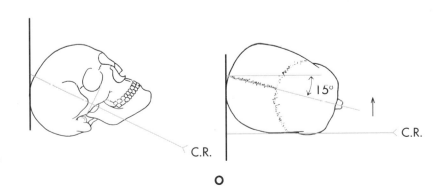

O

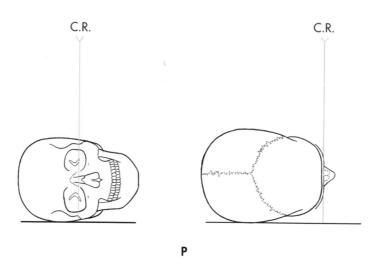

P

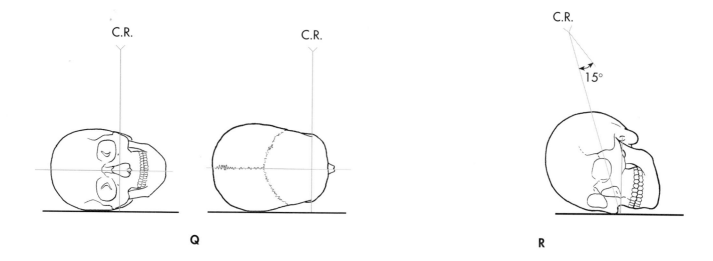

Q

R

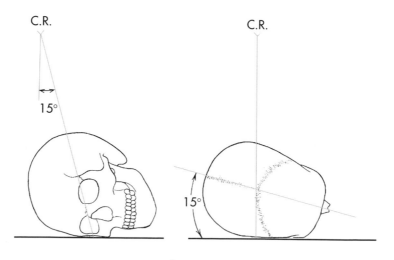

S

____ 1. AP axial (Towne method)

____ 2. PA axial (Haas method)

____ 3. PA axial (Caldwell method)

____ 4. parietoacanthial (Waters method)

____ 5. full basal projection of the cranium

____ 6. orbitoparietal oblique (Rhese method)

____ 7. PA to demonstrate sphenoidal sinuses

____ 8. parieto-orbital oblique (Rhese method)

____ 9. AP axial to demonstrate facial bones

____ 10. best projection to demonstrate maxillary sinuses

____ 11. demonstrates one temporomandibular joint

____ 12. axiolateral oblique (anterior profile; Arcelin method)

____ 13. axiolateral oblique (posterior profile; Stenvers method)

____ 14. shows a profile image of the pars petrosa closer to the film

____ 15. demonstrates the mastoid air cells of the side closer to the film

____ 16. orbitomeatal line should form an angle of 37 degrees with the film

____ 17. petrous ridges should be projected immediately below the maxillae

____ 18. lateral position and central ray alignment to demonstrate nasal bones

____ 19. lateral position and central ray alignment to demonstrate facial bones

____ 20. petrous ridges should be projected into the lower one-third of the orbits

____ 21. tangential projection to demonstrate individual zygomatic arches

____ 22. AP axial projection and central ray alignment to demonstrate bilateral zygomatic arches

____ 23. AP axial projection and central ray alignment to demonstrate temporomandibular joints

____ 24. produces a slightly oblique tangential image of one zygomatic arch free of superimposed shadows

____ 25. central ray should enter 2 inches (5 cm) posterior to and 2 inches (5 cm) above the uppermost external acoustic (auditory) meatus

Self-Test: Osteology, Arthrology, and Positioning of the Skull

Instructions: Answer the following questions by selecting the best choice.

1. What other term refers to the orbitomeatal line?

   a. acanthomeatal line
   b. glabellomeatal line
   c. radiographic base line
   d. base line of the cranium

2. Which positioning landmark is located at the base of the nasal spine?

   a. nasion
   b. gonion
   c. glabella
   d. acanthion

3. Which positioning landmark is located at the most superior point of the nasal bones?

   a. nasion
   b. canthus
   c. glabella
   d. acanthion

4. Which localization point is the smooth elevation located between the superciliary ridges?

   a. nasion
   b. glabella
   c. acanthion
   d. mental point

5. Which localization point is most superior?

   a. nasion
   b. gonion
   c. glabella
   d. acanthion

6. Where on the skull is the gonion located?

   a. between the orbits
   b. on the anterior frontal bone
   c. on the posterior occipital bone
   d. on the lateroposterior part of the mandible

7. Where on the skull is the outer canthus located?

   a. between the orbits
   b. at the mandibular angle
   c. along each parietal eminence
   d. on the lateral border of each orbit

8. Which positioning landmark is located at the anterior portion of the mandible?

   a. nasion
   b. gonion
   c. acanthion
   d. mental point

9. Which suture of the skull articulates the frontal bone with both parietal bones?

   a. coronal
   b. sagittal
   c. squamosal
   d. lambdoidal

10. Which suture of the skull joins both parietal bones at the vertex of the skull?

    a. coronal
    b. sagittal
    c. squamosal
    d. lambdoidal

11. Which suture of the skull joins a parietal bone with both a sphenoid bone and a temporal bone?

    a. coronal
    b. sagittal
    c. squamosal
    d. lambdoidal

12. Which suture of the skull joins both parietal bones with the occipital bone?

    a. coronal
    b. sagittal
    c. squamosal
    d. lambdoidal

13. The bregma fontanel is located at the junction of which two sutures?

    a. coronal and sagittal
    b. coronal and squamosal
    c. lambdoidal and sagittal
    d. lambdoidal and squamosal

14. The lambda fontanel is located at the junction of which two sutures?

    a. coronal and sagittal
    b. coronal and squamosal
    c. lambdoidal and sagittal
    d. lambdoidal and squamosal

15. The bregma fontanel is located at the junction of which cranial bones?

    a. frontal and both parietals
    b. occipital and both parietals
    c. frontal with both sphenoids and temporals
    d. occipital with both sphenoids and temporals

16. The lambda fontanel is located at the junction of which cranial bones?

    a. frontal and both parietals
    b. occipital and both parietals
    c. frontal with both sphenoids and temporals
    d. occipital with both sphenoids and temporals

17. Which skull classification refers to the typical skull in terms of width and length?

    a. mesocephalic
    b. brachycephalic
    c. dolichocephalic

18. Which skull classification refers to the long and narrow skull?

    a. mesocephalic
    b. brachycephalic
    c. dolichocephalic

19. Which skull classification refers to the short and wide skull?

    a. mesocephalic
    b. brachycephalic
    c. dolichocephalic

20. How many degrees from the median sagittal plane is the angle formed with the petrous pyramids in the mesocephalic skull?

    a. 36
    b. 40
    c. 47
    d. 54

21. How many degrees from the median sagittal plane is the angle formed with the petrous pyramids in the brachycephalic skull?

    a. 36
    b. 40
    c. 47
    d. 54

22. How many degrees from the median sagittal plane is the angle formed with the petrous pyramids in the dolichocephalic skull?

    a. 36
    b. 40
    c. 47
    d. 54

23. On which cranial bone are the superciliary ridges located?

    a. frontal
    b. ethmoid
    c. parietal
    d. occipital

24. On which cranial bone is the cribriform plate located?

    a. frontal
    b. ethmoid
    c. sphenoid
    d. temporal

25. On which cranial bone is the crista galli located?

    a. ethmoid
    b. temporal
    c. sphenoid
    d. occipital

26. Which cranial bone has a petrous pyramid?

    a. ethmoid
    b. sphenoid
    c. temporal
    d. parietal

27. On which cranial bone is the sella turcica located?

    a. frontal
    b. ethmoid
    c. temporal
    d. sphenoid

28. Which cranial bone has the mastoid process?

    a. ethmoid
    b. sphenoid
    c. parietal
    d. temporal

29. On which cranial bone is the perpendicular plate located?

    a. ethmoid
    b. sphenoid
    c. parietal
    d. temporal

30. Which cranial bone has both greater and lesser wings?

    a. ethmoid
    b. temporal
    c. sphenoid
    d. occipital

31. With which cranial bone does the first cervical vertebra articulate?

    a. ethmoid
    b. sphenoid
    c. temporal
    d. occipital

32. From which cranial bone do pterygoid processes project inferiorly?

    a. frontal
    b. ethmoid
    c. temporal
    d. sphenoid

33. Which cranial bone has the foramen magnum?

    a. frontal
    b. sphenoid
    c. temporal
    d. occipital

34. From which cranial bone does the zygomatic process arise?

    a. frontal
    b. temporal
    c. sphenoid
    d. parietal

35. The external acoustic (auditory) meatus is a part of which cranial bone?

    a. frontal
    b. temporal
    c. parietal
    d. sphenoid

36. Which term refers to the zygomatic bone?

    a. nasal
    b. malar
    c. vomer
    d. maxilla

37. Which bones comprise the bridge of the nose?

    a. nasal
    b. maxillae
    c. palatine
    d. lacrimal

38. In which bones are the antra of Highmore located?

    a. maxillae
    b. lacrimals
    c. zygomatics
    d. nasal conchae

39. Where are the lacrimal bones located?

    a. inside the nasal cavity
    b. on the medial wall of each orbit
    c. on the lateral wall of each orbit
    d. inferior to the maxillary sinuses

40. Where is the vomer bone found?

    a. on the floor of the nasal cavity
    b. on the lateral wall of the orbits
    c. posterior to the nasal bones
    d. in the posterior one-fourth of the roof of the mouth

41. Which bone comprises most of the lateral wall of the orbital cavities?

    a. maxilla
    b. zygomatic
    c. lacrimal
    d. palatine

42. Which term refers to the anterior process of the mandibular ramus?

    a. cornu
    b. condyle
    c. coracoid
    d. coronoid

43. Which term refers to the posterior process of the mandibular ramus?

    a. cornu
    b. condyle
    c. coronoid
    d. coracoid

44. Which facial bones have alveolar processes?

    a. vomer and mandible
    b. vomer and zygomatic
    c. maxillae and mandible
    d. maxillae and zygomatic

45. Which bones form the posterior one-fourth of the roof of the mouth?

    a. maxillae
    b. palatine
    c. zygomatic
    d. inferior nasal conchae

46. Which positioning landmark is located on the maxillae?

    a. gonion
    b. nasion
    c. acanthion
    d. mental point

47. Which two positioning lines/planes should be perpendicular to the film for the PA projection of the skull?

    a. orbitomeatal line and interpupillary line
    b. orbitomeatal line and median sagittal plane
    c. infraorbitomeatal line and interpupillary line
    d. infraorbitomeatal line and median sagittal plane

48. With reference to the patient, where should the film be centered for the PA projection of the skull?

    a. nasion
    b. glabella
    c. acanthion
    d. mental point

49. With reference to the patient, where should the film be centered for the lateral projection of the skull?

    a. nasion
    b. external acoustic (auditory) meatus
    c. 2 inches (5 cm) above the external acoustic (auditory) meatus
    d. 2 inches (5 cm) below the external acoustic (auditory) meatus

50. With reference to the film, how should the interpupillary line and the median sagittal plane be positioned for the lateral projection of the skull?

    a. interpupillary line, parallel; median sagittal plane, parallel
    b. interpupillary line, parallel; median sagittal plane, perpendicular
    c. interpupillary line, perpendicular; median sagittal plane, parallel
    d. interpupillary line, perpendicular; median sagittal plane, perpendicular

51. For the AP axial projection (Towne method) of the skull, how many degrees and in which direction should the central ray be directed when the orbitomeatal line is perpendicular to the film?

    a. 30 degrees caudad
    b. 30 degrees cephalad
    c. 37 degrees caudad
    d. 37 degrees cephalad

52. For the AP axial projection (Towne method) of the skull, how many degrees and in which direction should the central ray be directed when the infraorbitomeatal line is perpendicular to the film?

    a. 30 degrees caudad
    b. 30 degrees cephalad
    c. 37 degrees caudad
    d. 37 degrees cephalad

53. Which positioning line should be parallel with the film for the submentovertical projection of the skull?

    a. orbitomeatal line
    b. acanthomeatal line
    c. glabellomeatal line
    d. infraorbitomeatal line

54. Which projection of the skull can be correctly performed with the central ray angled 37 degrees?

    a. PA
    b. lateral
    c. submentovertical
    d. AP axial (Towne method)

55. Which projection of the skull can be correctly performed with the central ray angled 15 degrees?

    a. lateral
    b. submentovertical
    c. PA axial (Caldwell method)
    d. AP axial (Towne method)

56. Which evaluation criterion pertains to the AP axial projection (Towne method) of the skull?

    a. Orbital roofs should be superimposed.
    b. Mandibular symphysis should superimpose anterior frontal bone.
    c. Part of the sella turcica should be seen within the foramen magnum.
    d. Distance from the lateral border of the skull to the lateral border of the orbit should be the same on both sides.

57. Which evaluation criterion pertains to the PA projection of the skull?

    a. Orbital roofs should be superimposed.
    b. Mandibular symphysis should superimpose anterior frontal bone.
    c. Part of the sella turcica should be seen within the foramen magnum.
    d. Distance from the lateral border of the skull to the lateral border of the orbit should be the same on both sides.

58. Which evaluation criterion pertains to the lateral projection of the skull?

    a. Orbital roofs should be superimposed.
    b. Mandibular symphysis should superimpose anterior frontal bone.
    c. Part of the sella turcica should be seen within the foramen magnum.
    d. Distance from the lateral border of the skull to the lateral border of the orbit should be the same on both sides.

59. Which evaluation criterion pertains to the submentovertical projection of the skull?

    a. Orbital roofs should be superimposed.
    b. Mandibular symphysis should superimpose anterior frontal bone.
    c. Part of the sella turcica should be seen within the foramen magnum.
    d. Distance from the lateral border of the skull to the lateral border of the orbit should be the same on both sides.

60. Which projection of the skull produces a full basal image of the cranium?

    a. lateral
    b. AP axial (Towne method)
    c. submentovertical (Schüller method)
    d. PA with perpendicular central ray

61. For the PA axial projection (Haas method) of the skull, where should the central ray enter the patient's head?

    a. nasion
    b. acanthion
    c. 11/2 inches (3.7 cm) above the external occipital protuberance
    d. 11/2 inches (3.7 cm) below the external occipital protuberance

62. How many degrees and in which direction should the central ray be directed for the PA axial projection (Haas method) of the skull?

    a. 15 degrees caudad
    b. 15 degrees cephalad
    c. 25 degrees caudad
    d. 25 degrees cephalad

63. For the parieto-orbital oblique projection (Rhese method) of the skull, which positioning line should be perpendicular to the film?

    a. orbitomeatal
    b. acanthomeatal
    c. glabellomeatal
    d. infraorbitomeatal

64. For the orbitoparietal oblique projection (Rhese method) of the skull, which positioning line should be perpendicular to the film?

    a. infraorbitomeatal
    b. glabellomeatal
    c. acanthomeatal
    d. orbitomeatal

65. With reference to the orbit, where should the optic foramen be imaged on the radiograph to indicate correct positioning of the patient for the parieto-orbital oblique projection (Rhese method) of the skull?

    a. within the lower inner quadrant
    b. within the lower outer quadrant
    c. within the upper inner quadrant
    d. within the upper outer quadrant

66. For the parieto-orbital oblique projection (Rhese method) of the skull, an angle of how many degrees should be formed between the median sagittal plane and the film?

    a. 25
    b. 37
    c. 53
    d. 55

67. With reference to the film, how should the interpupillary line and the median sagittal plane be positioned for the lateral projection to demonstrate the sella turcica?

    a. interpupillary line, parallel; median sagittal plane, parallel
    b. interpupillary line, parallel; median sagittal plane, perpendicular
    c. interpupillary line, perpendicular; median sagittal plane, parallel
    d. interpupillary line, perpendicular; median sagittal plane, perpendicular

68. For the lateral projection to demonstrate the sella turcica, where should the central ray be directed?

    a. 3/4 inch (1.9 cm) anterior and 3/4 inch (1.9 cm) inferior to the external acoustic (auditory) meatus
    b. 3/4 inch (1.9 cm) anterior and 3/4 inch (1.9 cm) superior to the external acoustic (auditory) meatus
    c. 3/4 inch (1.9 cm) posterior and 3/4 inch (1.9 cm) inferior to the external acoustic (auditory) meatus
    d. 3/4 inch (1.9 cm) posterior and 3/4 inch (1.9 cm) superior to the external acoustic (auditory) meatus

69. With reference to the patient, where should the central ray be directed for the lateral projection of the facial bones?

    a. zygoma
    b. nasal bones
    c. outer canthus
    d. 3/4 inch (1.9 cm) anterior and 3/4 inch (1.9 cm) superior to the external acoustic (auditory) meatus

70. Which positioning line and angle indicate correct positioning of the head for the parietoacanthial projection (Waters method)?

    a. orbitomeatal line 37 degrees to the film
    b. orbitomeatal line perpendicular to the film
    c. infraorbitomeatal line 37 degrees to the film
    d. infraorbitomeatal line perpendicular to the film

71. Which evaluation criterion pertains to the parietoacanthial projection (Waters method)?

    a. Orbital roofs should be superimposed.
    b. Petrous ridges should be projected within the orbits.
    c. Zygomatic arches should be free from overlying structures.
    d. Petrous ridges should be projected immediately below the maxillae.

72. Which evaluation criterion pertains to the lateral projection of the facial bones?

    a. Orbital roofs should be superimposed.
    b. Petrous ridges should be projected within the orbits.
    c. Zygomatic arches should be free from overlying structures.
    d. Petrous ridges should be projected immediately below the maxillae.

73. Which evaluation criterion pertains to the tangential (basal) projection for bilateral zygomatic arches?

    a. Orbital roofs should be superimposed.
    b. Zygomatic arches should be superimposed.
    c. Petrous ridges should be projected within the orbits.
    d. Zygomatic arches should be free from overlying structures.

74. Which evaluation criterion pertains to the parietoacanthial projection (Waters method)?

    a. Orbital roofs should be superimposed.
    b. Zygomatic arches should be superimposed.
    c. Petrous pyramids should be projected within the orbits.
    d. Distance between the lateral border of the skull and orbit should be the same on both sides.

75. An AP axial projection for bilateral zygomatic arches produces an image similar to the AP axial projection (Towne method) of the skull. How many degrees and in which direction should the central ray be directed for this projection to demonstrate zygomatic arches?

    a. 30 degrees caudad
    b. 37 degrees caudad
    c. 30 degrees cephalad
    d. 37 degrees cephalad

76. An AP axial projection for bilateral zygomatic arches is performed similarly to the AP axial projection (Towne method) of the skull except that the projection for zygomatic arches requires that the:

   a. central ray be directed cephalically.
   b. central ray be directed to the glabella.
   c. orbitomeatal line form an angle of 37 degrees with the film.
   d. median sagittal plane form an angle of 45 degrees with the film.

77. With reference to the film, how should the median sagittal plane be adjusted for the tangential projection to demonstrate an individual zygomatic arch?

   a. parallel with the film
   b. angled 37 degrees to the film
   c. angled 53 degrees to the film
   d. moved 15 degrees from perpendicular

78. How many degrees and in which direction should the central ray be directed for the axiolateral oblique projection of the mandible?

   a. 25 degrees caudad
   b. 25 degrees cephalad
   c. 37 degrees caudad
   d. 37 degrees cephalad

79. Which structures are best demonstrated with an axiolateral oblique projection?

   a. facial bones
   b. zygomatic arches
   c. maxillary sinuses
   d. temporomandibular joints

80. How many degrees and in which direction should the central ray be directed for the axiolateral oblique projection for TMJs?

   a. 15 degrees caudad
   b. 15 degrees cephalad
   c. 25 degrees caudad
   d. 25 degrees cephalad

81. For the AP axial projection for TMJs, where should the central ray be directed?

   a. nasion
   b. glabella
   c. acanthion
   d. 3 inches (7.5 cm) above the nasion

82. With reference to the patient, where should the film be centered for the axiolateral oblique projection for TMJs?

   a. to the glabella
   b. 1/2 inch (1.2 cm) anterior to the external acoustic (auditory) meatus
   c. 1 inch (2.5 cm) posterior to the external acoustic (auditory) meatus
   d. 2 inches (5 cm) above the external acoustic (auditory) meatus

83. To demonstrate the posterior two-thirds of the mandibular body with the patient positioned semisupine for the axiolateral oblique projection, the head should be resting on the:

   a. cheek.
   b. tip of the nose.
   c. mental symphysis.
   d. side of the chin.

84. How many degrees and in which direction should the central ray be directed for the axiolateral oblique projection of the mandible?

   a. 20 degrees caudad
   b. 20 degrees cephalad
   c. 30 degrees caudad
   d. 30 degrees cephalad

85. Which projection requires the patient's head to be placed on a cranially inclined cassette, elevating the edge of the cassette closest to the shoulder?

   a. axiolateral oblique
   b. axiolateral (Law method)
   c. axiolateral oblique (anterior profile; Arcelin method)
   d. axiolateral oblique (posterior profile; Stenvers method)

86. Which evaluation criterion pertains to the axiolateral oblique projection of the mandible?

   a. Mandibular rami should be superimposed.
   b. Mandibular condyles should be anterior to the petrous ridges.
   c. Opposite side of the mandible should not superimpose the body.
   d. Mandibular symphysis should superimpose anterior frontal bone.

87. For the modified Caldwell method of the PA axial projection for sinuses, in addition to the median sagittal plane, which positioning line should be perpendicular to the film?

   a. orbitomeatal
   b. glabellomeatal
   c. interpupillary
   d. infraorbitomeatal

88. Which sinus groups are best demonstrated with the PA axial projection (Caldwell method)?

    a. frontal and sphenoidal
    b. frontal and anterior ethmoidal
    c. maxillary and sphenoidal
    d. maxillary and anterior ethmoidal

89. How many degrees and in which direction should the central ray be directed for the modified Caldwell method of the PA axial projection for sinuses?

    a. 15 degrees caudad
    b. 15 degrees cephalad
    c. 23 degrees caudad
    d. 23 degrees cephalad

90. Where should petrous ridges be seen in the image of the PA axial projection (Caldwell method) for paranasal sinuses?

    a. superior to the orbits
    b. lower one-third of the orbits
    c. below the maxillary sinuses
    d. through the maxillary sinuses

91. For the original Caldwell method of the PA axial projection for sinuses, in addition to the median sagittal plane, which positioning line should be perpendicular to the film?

    a. orbitomeatal
    b. acanthomeatal
    c. glabellomeatal
    d. infraorbitomeatal

92. How many degrees and in which direction should the central ray be directed for the original Caldwell method of the PA axial projection for paranasal sinuses?

    a. 15 degrees caudad
    b. 15 degrees cephalad
    c. 23 degrees caudad
    d. 23 degrees cephalad

93. With reference to the patient, where should the film be centered for the PA axial projection (Caldwell method)?

    a. nasion
    b. acanthion
    c. mental point
    d. 3 inches (7.5 cm) above the nasion

94. With reference to the outer canthus, where should the film be centered for the lateral projection for sinuses?

    a. anterior
    b. posterior
    c. superior
    d. inferior

95. Which sinus group is of primary importance in the lateral view of the sinuses?

    a. frontal
    b. ethmoidal
    c. sphenoidal
    d. maxillary

96. Which positioning line should form an angle of 37 degrees with the film for the parietoacanthial projection (Waters method)?

    a. orbitomeatal
    b. acanthomeatal
    c. glabellomeatal
    d. infraorbitomeatal

97. With reference to the film, how should the central ray be directed for the parietoacanthial projection (Waters method)?

    a. perpendicular
    b. 15 degrees caudad
    c. 23 degrees caudad
    d. 37 degrees caudad

98. Which paranasal sinus group is best demonstrated with the parietoacanthial projection (Waters method)?

    a. frontal
    b. ethmoidal
    c. sphenoidal
    d. maxillary

99. Where should the petrous ridges be seen in the image of the parietoacanthial projection for paranasal sinuses?

    a. superior to the orbits
    b. lower one-third of the orbits
    c. below the maxillary sinuses
    d. through the maxillary sinuses

100. With reference to the patient, where should the film be centered for the parietoacanthial projection (Waters method)?

    a. nasion
    b. glabella
    c. acanthion
    d. mental point

101. Which two paranasal sinus groups are better demonstrated with the submentovertical projection than are the other sinuses?

    a. ethmoidal and sphenoidal
    b. ethmoidal and maxillary
    c. frontal and sphenoidal
    d. frontal and maxillary

102. Which projection of the paranasal sinuses is a basal projection?

    a. lateral
    b. submentovertical
    c. PA axial (Caldwell method)
    d. parietoacanthial (Waters method)

103. Which evaluation criterion pertains to the lateral projection for paranasal sinuses?

    a. All four sinus groups should be included.
    b. Petrous pyramids should lie in the lower one-third of the orbits.
    c. Mandibular symphysis should superimpose anterior frontal bone.
    d. Petrous pyramids should lie immediately below the floor of the maxillary sinuses.

104. Which evaluation criterion pertains to the lateral projection for paranasal sinuses?

    a. Orbital roofs should be superimposed.
    b. Petrous ridges should lie in the lower one-third of the orbits.
    c. Mandibular condyles should be anterior to the petrous ridges.
    d. Mandibular symphysis should superimpose anterior frontal bone.

105. Which evaluation criterion pertains to the PA axial projection (Caldwell method) for sinuses?

    a. All four sinus groups should be included.
    b. Frontal and ethmoidal sinuses should be seen.
    c. Mandibular condyles should be anterior to the petrous ridges.
    d. Petrous ridges should lie immediately below the floor of the maxillary sinuses.

106. Which evaluation criterion pertains to the PA axial projection (Caldwell method) for paranasal sinuses?

    a. Orbital roofs should be superimposed.
    b. Mandibular rami should be superimposed.
    c. Petrous ridges should lie in the lower one-third of the orbits.
    d. Petrous ridges should lie immediately below the floor of the maxillary sinuses.

107. Which evaluation criterion pertains to the parietoacanthial projection (Waters method) for paranasal sinuses?

    a. Mandibular rami should be superimposed.
    b. Petrous ridges should lie in the lower one-third of the orbits.
    c. Mandibular symphysis should superimpose anterior frontal bone.
    d. Petrous ridges should lie immediately below the floor of the maxillary sinuses.

108. Which evaluation criterion pertains to the submentovertical projection for paranasal sinuses?

    a. Mandibular rami should be superimposed.
    b. Frontal and ethmoidal sinuses should be clearly seen.
    c. Mandibular symphysis should superimpose anterior frontal bone.
    d. Petrous ridges should lie immediately below the floor of the maxillary sinuses.

109. Which evaluation criterion pertains to the submentovertical projection for sinuses?

    a. Petrous ridges should lie in the lower one-third of the orbits.
    b. Mandibular condyles should be anterior to the petrous ridges.
    c. Mandibular condyles should be posterior to the petrous ridges.
    d. Petrous ridges should lie immediately below the floor of the maxillary sinuses.

110. Which sinus group is not well demonstrated in the image produced by the parietoacanthial projection (Waters method)?

   a. ethmoidal
   b. frontal
   c. sphenoidal
   d. maxillary

111. Which structures should always be radiographed with the patient in an upright position?

   a. orbits
   b. mastoids
   c. zygomatic arches
   d. paranasal sinuses

112. What is the only projection for paranasal sinuses that adequately demonstrates all four sinus groups?

   a. lateral
   b. submentovertical
   c. PA axial (Caldwell method)
   d. parietoacanthial (Waters method)

113. Which projection method produces an axiolateral view of a mastoid?

   a. Law method
   b. Waters method
   c. Arcelin method
   d. Stenvers method

114. Which projection requires the central ray to be directed 15 degrees caudad?

   a. axiolateral (Law method)
   b. parietoacanthial (Waters method)
   c. axiolateral oblique (anterior profile; Arcelin method)
   d. axiolateral oblique (posterior profile; Stenvers method)

115. Which projection requires the patient's head to be rotated from true lateral, moving the face closer to the film until the median sagittal plane forms an angle of 15 degrees with the film?

   a. axiolateral (Law method)
   b. parietoacanthial (Waters method)
   c. axiolateral oblique (anterior profile; Arcelin method)
   d. axiolateral oblique (posterior profile; Stenvers method)

116. For the single tube-angulation method for the axiolateral projection (Law method), how many degrees and in which direction should the central ray be directed?

   a. 10 degrees caudad
   b. 10 degrees cephalad
   c. 15 degrees caudad
   d. 15 degrees cephalad

117. How many degrees and in which direction should the central ray be directed for the axiolateral oblique projection (posterior profile; Stenvers method)?

   a. 10 degrees caudad
   b. 10 degrees cephalad
   c. 12 degrees caudad
   d. 12 degrees cephalad

118. How many degrees and in which direction should the central ray be directed for the axiolateral oblique projection (anterior profile; Arcelin method)?

   a. 10 degrees caudad
   b. 10 degrees cephalad
   c. 12 degrees caudad
   d. 12 degrees cephalad

119. Which evaluation criterion pertains to the axiolateral projection (Law method)?

   a. Petrous ridges should lie in the lower one-third of both orbits.
   b. Petrous ridges should be demonstrated in profile without distortion.
   c. Mastoid process should be projected below the shadow of the occipital bone.
   d. Mastoid closer to the film should be included, with the air cells demonstrated and centered to the film.

120. Which evaluation criterion pertains to the axiolateral oblique projection (posterior profile; Stenvers method)?

   a. Petrous ridge should lie in the lower one-third of the orbit.
   b. Petrous ridge should be demonstrated in profile without distortion.
   c. Mastoid process should be projected below the shadow of the occipital bone.
   d. Mastoid closer to the film should be included, with the air cells demonstrated and centered to the film.

121. Which projection requires the patient's head to be rotated from the PA position until the median sagittal plane forms an angle of 45 degrees with the film and the central ray to be directed to exit the skull 1 inch (2.5 cm) anterior to the external acoustic (auditory) meatus?

a. axiolateral (Law method)
b. tangential for individual zygomatic arches
c. axiolateral oblique (anterior profile; Arcelin method)
d. axiolateral oblique (posterior profile; Stenvers method)

122. Which structures are best demonstrated when the patient's head is rotated from true lateral, moving the face closer to the film until the median sagittal plane forms an angle of 15 degrees with the plane of the film, and the central ray is directed caudally to exit the skull 1 inch (2.5 cm) posterior to the external acoustic (auditory) meatus?

a. zygomatic arches
b. petrous portions
c. mastoid air cells
d. temporomandibular joints

123. Which projection requires the patient's head to be rotated from the AP position until the median sagittal plane forms an angle of 45 degrees with the plane of the film and the central ray to be directed to enter the side of the face at a point about 1 inch (2.5 cm) anterior and 3/4 inch (1.9 cm) superior to the external acoustic (auditory) meatus?

a. axiolateral (Law method)
b. submentovertical (Schüller method)
c. axiolateral oblique (anterior profile; Arcelin method)
d. axiolateral oblique (posterior profile; Stenvers method)

124. Which structure is best demonstrated when the patient's head is rotated from the PA position, moving the occipital bone closer to the right shoulder until the median sagittal plane forms an angle of 45 degrees with the plane of the film, and the central ray is directed to exit the skull 1 inch (2.5 cm) anterior to the external acoustic (auditory) meatus?

a. left petrous portion
b. right petrous portion
c. left mastoid air cells
d. right mastoid air cells

125. Which structure is best demonstrated when the patient's head is rotated from the AP position, moving the face toward the right shoulder until the median sagittal plane forms an angle of 45 degrees with the plane of the film, and the central ray is directed to enter the side of the face about 1 inch (2.5 cm) anterior and 3/4 inch (1.9 cm) superior to the external acoustic (auditory) meatus?

a. left petrous portion
b. right petrous portion
c. left mastoid air cells
d. right mastoid air cells

Volume 2
ANSWERS TO EXERCISES

Chapter 14: **Mouth and Salivary Glands**

Chapter 14 Review

1. A. posterior arch
   B. anterior arch
   C. tonsil
   D. hard palate
   E. uvula
   F. soft palate
   G. faucial isthmus
   H. tongue
2. A. orifice of submandibular (submaxillary) duct
   B. tongue
   C. frenulum of tongue
   D. sublingual fold
3. A. parotid (Stensen's) duct
   B. sublingual ducts (ducts of Rivinus)
   C. submandibular (Wharton's) duct
   D. sublingual gland
   E. parotid gland
   F. submandibular (submaxillary) gland
4. A. muscle tissue
   B. ramus of mandible
   C. parotid gland
   D. tongue
   E. dens
   F. atlas
   G. spinal cord
5. A. mandible
   B. oropharynx
   C. cervical vertebral body
   D. sublingual gland
   E. submandibular (submaxillary) gland
   F. tip of parotid gland
6. mouth
7. the process of chewing and grinding food into small pieces
8. teeth
9. to soften food, keep the mouth moist, and contribute digestive enzymes
10. parotid, sublingual, and submandibular (submaxillary)
11. 1. b
    2. c
    3. a
12. Bartholin's
13. sublingual
14. radiographic examination of the salivary glands and ducts with the use of a contrast medium
15. computed tomography and magnetic resonance imaging
16. water-soluble, iodinated
17. because salivary gland pairs are in close proximity
18. to detect any condition demonstrable without the use of a contrast medium and to establish the optimal exposure factors
19. to open a duct for ready identification of its orifice and for easier passage of a cannula or catheter
20. tangential, lateral, and axial (intraoral method)
21. parotid
22. lateral
23. True
24. True
25. False. Only one parotid gland can be demonstrated with each tangential projection.
26. parotid
27. submandibular
28. to displace the submandibular gland below the mandible
29. sublingual and submandibular
30. axial (intraoral method)
31. axial (intraoral method)
32. tangential
33. a. tangential
    b. parotid
    c. Fill the mouth with air and then puff the cheeks out as much as possible.
34. a. lateral
    b. parotid
    c. parotid (Stensen's)
35. a. lateral
    b. submandibular
    c. submandibular (Wharton's)

Self-Test: Mouth and Salivary Glands

1. a	6. d
2. a	7. c
3. c	8. b
4. a	9. c
5. a	10. a

Chapter 15: **Anterior Part of the Neck**

Chapter 15 Review

1. A. nasal septum
   B. nasopharynx
   C. uvula
   D. vallecula epiglottica
   E. epiglottis
   F. vocal folds
   G. larynx
   H. laryngopharynx
   I. soft palate
   J. median glossoepiglottic fold
   K. piriform recess (sinus)
   L. rima glottidis
2. A. soft palate
   B. nasopharynx
   C. uvula
   D. oropharynx
   E. vallecula epiglottica
   F. epiglottis
   G. false vestibular folds (false vocal folds)
   H. vocal folds

I. larynx
J. hard palate
K. ventricle
L. laryngopharynx
M. trachea
N. esophagus
3. A. inferior constrictor muscle
B. superior thyroid artery
C. superior parathyroid gland
D. inferior constrictor muscle
E. thyroid gland
F. inferior thyroid artery
G. inferior parathyroid gland
H. esophagus
I. thyroid cartilage
J. cricothyroid ligament
K. isthmus of thyroid
L. trachea
M. recurrent laryngeal nerve
4. A. hyoid bone
B. thyroid cartilage
C. cricothyroid ligament
D. cricoid cartilage
E. trachea
5. A. base of tongue
B. epiglottis
C. vestibular fold
D. rima glottidis (open)
E. rima glottidis (closed)
F. vocal chords
G. vallecula epiglottica
H. lateral glossoepiglottic fold
I. median glossoepiglottic fold
6. posterior; anterior
7. trachea
8. esophagus
9. thyroid; parathyroid
10. pharynx
11. nasopharynx
12. oropharynx
13. larynx
14. glottis
15. AP; lateral
16. breathing, phonation, stress maneuvers, and swallowing
17. a. supine
    b. upright
18. laryngeal prominence
19. a. level of the external acoustic meatuses
    b. level of the mandibular angles
    c. level of the laryngeal prominence
20. A. air-filled pharynx
    B. hyoid bone
    C. laryngeal structures
    D. trachea

Self-Test: Anterior Part of the Neck

1. a	6. d
2. a	7. c
3. c	8. b
4. b	9. b
5. b	10. b

Chapter 16: The Digestive System: Abdomen, Liver, Spleen, and Biliary Tract
Part 1: Anatomy of the Abdomen, the Liver, the Spleen, and the Biliary Tract

Exercise 1

1. A. right lobe of the liver
B. liver
C. gall bladder
D. ascending colon
E. ileum
F. cecum
G. appendix
H. left lobe of the liver
I. pancreas
J. esophagus
K. stomach
L. spleen
M. left colic splenic flexure
N. descending colon
O. transverse colon
P. small intestine
Q. sigmoid colon
R. urinary bladder
2. A. tongue
B. sublingual gland
C. submandibular (submaxillary) gland
D. gall bladder
E. biliary ducts
F. visceral surface of the liver
G. appendix
H. parotid gland
I. pharynx
J. esophagus
K. stomach
L. spleen
M. pancreas
N. large intestine
O. small intestine
3. A. hepatopancreatic ampulla
B. cystic duct
C. right lobe of the liver
D. gall bladder
E. liver
F. falciform ligament

G. quadrate lobe of the liver
H. left lobe of the liver
I. left hepatic duct
J. caudate lobe of the liver
K. common hepatic duct
L. common bile duct
M. pancreatic duct
N. pancreas
O. duodenum
4. A. cut surface of liver
   B. gall bladder
   C. cystic duct
   D. right kidney
   E. common hepatic duct
   F. common bile duct
   G. spleen
   H. left kidney
   I. pancreas
   J. duodenum
5. A. liver
   B. inferior vena cava
   C. right kidney
   D. stomach
   E. spleen
   F. left kidney
   G. aorta

Exercise 2

1. peritoneum
2. parietal and visceral
3. parietal
4. visceral
5. liver
6. liver
7. bile
8. common hepatic duct
9. gall bladder
10. liver
11. True
12. False. The gall bladder is located on the inferior surface of the right lobe of the liver, within the abdominal cavity.
13. common bile duct
14. pancreatic duct
15. cholecystokinin
16. hepatopancreatic ampulla
17. pancreas
18. True
19. True
20. True

Part 2: **Positioning of the Abdomen and Gall Bladder**

Exercise 1 Positioning for the Abdomen

1. KUB
2. iliac crests

3. 2 to 3 inches (5 to 7.5 cm) above the iliac crests, or high enough to include the diaphragm; and to the level of the iliac crests, to include the bladder
4. Gonadal shielding is desirable if the gonads lie within close proximity (2 inches [5 cm]) to the primary x-ray field. Gonadal shielding should be used if the clinical objectives of the examination will not be compromised. Gonadal shielding should be used if the patient has a reasonable reproductive potential.
5. 70
6. exhalation; to elevate the diaphragm to its highest point and thus relax the abdominal viscera
7. to allow the patient to come to rest and to allow the involuntary movement of the viscera to subside
8. True
9. Spinous processes should be in the center of the lumbar vertebrae. If seen, ischial spines of the pelvis should be symmetric. Alae or wings of the ilia should be symmetric.
10. diaphragm; to demonstrate any free air within the abdominal cavity that may rise and become trapped under the diaphragm
11. a right or left marker and an appropriate marker indicating the patient is upright
12. a reduction in the radiation exposure to the gonads
13. supine KUB, AP upright abdomen, and PA chest
14. to demonstrate abdominal free air that may accumulate under the diaphragm
15. left lateral decubitus
16. demonstration of air-fluid levels
17. to enable rising free air to be seen through the homogeneous background density of the liver instead of becoming superimposed with air in the stomach
18. The patient should be recumbent in a lateral position with the left side down (left lateral recumbent), both arms raised above the diaphragm, and the knees slightly flexed.
19. A vertically placed cassette should be centered against the patient's posterior side of the abdomen at the level of the iliac crests.
20. Suspend respiration after exhalation.
21. perpendicularly (horizontally) to the midpoint of the cassette, entering at the level of the iliac crests
22. the side that is up
23. the dependent (down) side
24. diaphragm
25. markers indicating the side of the patient and which side is up
26. AP projection with the patient in the left lateral decubitus position
27. True
28. False. Make the exposure after the patient suspends respiration after exhalation.
29. iliac crests, or high enough to ensure demonstrating the diaphragm
30. across the pelvis
31. to a point on the median coronal plane at the level of the iliac crests

32. pelvis and lumbar vertebrae
33. right lateral recumbent
34. Lateral projection with the patient in the dorsal decubitus position
35. median coronal plane
36. 2 inches (5 cm)
37. to relieve strain on the patient's back; it reduces the lordotic curvature
38. exhalation
39. True
40. Diaphragm should be included without motion.
    Abdominal contents should be seen with soft tissue gray tones.
    The entire abdomen should be demonstrated.

Exercise 2 Contrast Studies for the Gall Bladder

1. cholecystography
2. oral
3. OCG; GB
4. portal
5. a. its ability to remove the contrast medium from blood and excrete it with the bile
   b. their patency and condition
   c. the concentrating and emptying ability, thus the presence of neoplasms and calculi
6. gallstones
7. True
8. True
9. preliminary preparation of the intestinal tract; preliminary diet; exact time to swallow the oral tablets; avoidance of laxatives for 24 hours before swallowing the tablets; avoidance of all foods, both solids and liquids (except water) after swallowing the tablets; and the time to report for the examination
10. Vomiting or diarrhea may cause most of the contrast medium to be expelled from the patient, rendering a poorly and partially opacified gall bladder.
11. Prolonged fasting can cause the formation of gas, which could make it difficult to clearly visualize the gall bladder.
12. Preparation for the OCG can be shortened if the intestinal tract is found to be sufficiently clean; and radiopaque gallstones may be demonstrated before they can be obscured by the contrast medium.
13. The intestinal tract needs 24 hours to allow irritation of the mucosal lining to subside and to prevent the egestion of the contrast medium with the fecal material.
14. only small drinks of water
15. ultrasonography
16. True
17. False. The right side of the abdomen should be centered to the midline of the table.
18. small
19. 1/2 second
20. Have the patient spread the breasts superiorly and laterally to clear the gall bladder region.

21. to rotate the vertebrae slightly to the left
22. Elevate the ankles.
23. exhalation
24. 2; to permit any peristaltic action to subside and to give the patient time to relax
25. a. Figure 16-8
    b. Figure 16-9
26. Make the exposure after the patient suspends respiration after inhalation.
27. a. sthenic
    b. hypersthenic
    c. asthenic
28. lower
29. 2 to 4 inches (5 to 10 cm)
30. fundic
31. a. P
    b. P
    c. U
    d. U
    e. P
    f. U
    g. U
    h. U
32. vertebral column (vertebrae or thoracic vertebrae are also acceptable)
33. 15 to 40
34. the location of the gall bladder with reference to the vertebral column; the angulation of the long axis of the gall bladder; and whether the right colic (hepatic) flexure is clear or obscures the gall bladder
35. thin patients
36. The LAO position places the gall bladder closer to the film.
37. to compress the viscera and thus help eliminate movement
38. Because the gall bladder is normally on the right side of the abdomen, a right lateral position places the gall bladder closer to the film than does a left lateral. (A left lateral position should be the lateral of choice if the patient has the gall bladder on the left side of the abdomen.)
39. renal (kidney)
40. exhalation
41. thin
42. short
43. True
44. False. The mobility of the gall bladder often causes the organ to partially superimpose the vertebrae when the patient is placed in the left lateral position, thus making it difficult to clearly completely image the gall bladder without bony superimposition.
45. a. left anterior oblique
    b. right lateral decubitus
    c. PA (prone)
    d. PA (upright)

Self-Test: The Abdomen and the Gall Bladder

1. a	14. a	27. b	40. a
2. d	15. d	28. a	41. b
3. d	16. b	29. a	42. a
4. b	17. d	30. d	43. b
5. c	18. a	31. d	44. a
6. c	19. d	32. d	45. c
7. b	20. c	33. b	46. a
8. c	21. a	34. b	47. d
9. a	22. b	35. d	48. d
10. d	23. c	36. a	49. c
11. b	24. a	37. b	50. d
12. b	25. a	38. b	
13. a	26. a	39. a	

Chapter 17: **The Digestive System: The Alimentary Tract**
Part 1: **Anatomy of the Alimentary Tract**

Exercise 1

1. A. tongue
   B. sublingual gland
   C. submandibular gland
   D. gall bladder
   E. biliary ducts
   F. (visceral surface of) liver
   G. (posterior surface of) liver
   H. appendix
   I. parotid gland
   J. pharynx
   K. esophagus
   L. stomach
   M. spleen
   N. pancreas
   O. large intestine
   P. small intestine
2. A. cardiac antrum
   B. lesser curvature
   C. angular notch
   D. pyloric sphincter
   E. duodenum
   F. pyloric canal (antrum)
   G. sulcus intermedius
   H. pyloric antrum (vestibule)
   I. greater curvature
   J. cardiac notch
   K. fundus
   L. body
3. A. cardiac sphincter
   B. pyloric sphincter
   C. duodenum
   D. pyloric canal
   E. gastric folds (rugae)

4. A. greater duodenal papilla (orifice of biliary and pancreatic ducts)
   B. hepatopancreatic ampulla (ampulla of Vater)
   C. gall bladder
   D. cystic duct
   E. common hepatic duct
   F. common bile duct
   G. pylorus
   H. stomach
   I. pancreatic duct
   J. pancreas
   K. duodenum
5. A. ileum
   B. appendix
   C. cecum
   D. ascending colon
   E. right colic (hepatic) flexure
   F. transverse colon
   G. left colic (splenic) flexure
   H. descending colon
   I. sigmoid colon
   J. rectum
   K. urinary bladder
6. A. rectal ampulla
   B. sacrum
   C. anal canal

Exercise 2

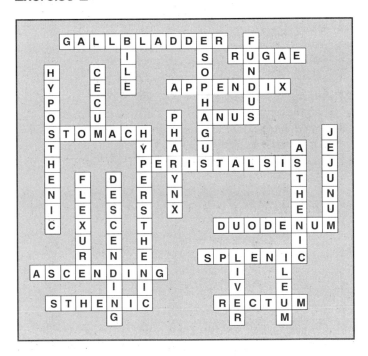

Exercise 3

1. b
2. a
3. c
4. b

5. a
6. c
7. a
8. b
9. a
10. c
11. b
12. c
13. c
14. c
15. c
16. b
17. a
18. a
19. a
20. c

Exercise 4

1. esophagus
2. cardiac antrum
3. cardiac orifice
4. stomach
5. rugae
6. right (medial)
7. pylorus
8. greater curvature
9. a. hypersthenic
   b. sthenic
   c. hyposthenic
   d. asthenic
10. cardia, fundus, body, and pylorus
11. cardia
12. fundus
13. pyloric
14. pyloric orifice
15. duodenum, jejunum, and ileum
16. duodenum
17. duodenal bulb
18. ileocecal valve
19. duodenum
20. jejunum
21. ileum
22. duodenum; ileum
23. small intestine
24. ileocecal valve
25. cecum
26. cecum
27. right colic flexure
28. ascending colon
29. transverse colon
30. left colic flexure
31. descending colon
32. descending colon and rectum
33. rectum
34. anal canal
35. anus

Part 2: **Positioning of the Alimentary Tract**

Exercise 1 Positioning for the Esophagus

1. True
2. True
3. False. A 30 to 50% weight/volume suspension is acceptable. The most important criterion for the barium is that it must flow sufficiently to coat esophageal walls.
4. a high-density barium product and carbon dioxide crystals
5. AP (or PA), oblique (RAO or LPO), and lateral
6. The LAO position may superimpose vertebral shadows with the distal esophagus.
7. T5 to T6
8. RAO and LPO
9. 35; 45
10. It allows more complete contrast filling of the esophagus.
11. The esophagus should be adequately demonstrated through the superimposed thoracic vertebrae.
12. to the left of the vertebral column, between the thoracic vertebrae and the heart
13. partially obscured by thoracic vertebrae
14. Posterior ribs should be superimposed.
15. cardiac orifice

Exercise 2 The Gastrointestinal Series

1. GI and UGI
2. to reduce the production of intestinal gas and fecal material
3. The coating ability of the barium may be diminished because the secretion of gastric juices may be stimulated.
4. a barium sulfate product of 30 to 50% weight/volume concentration
5. single-contrast examination and double-contrast examination
6. 30 to 50%
7. high-density barium sulfate suspension and gas-producing substance
8. Small lesions are readily demonstrated, and mucosal lining of the stomach can be more clearly visualized.
9. False. The examination should begin with the patient upright.
10. True
11. False. Most radiographs are obtained with the patient recumbent to provide better coating of the mucosal surface.
12. to coat the mucosal lining of the stomach
13. It relaxes the gastric tract, enabling gastric structures to expand and become better demonstrated.
14. The patient should be asked not to belch.
15. a UGI examination in which the patient is first examined with the double-contrast procedure, after which a low weight/volume barium sulfate suspension is given and the patient is then examined with the single-contrast procedure
16. double-contrast
17. with intubation and without intubation
18. True
19. True

20. True
21. False. The patient should be in the recumbent position.
22. True
23. True
24. False. A compression band should not be used for immobilizing the patient, because its use can cause filling defects and interfere with the filling and emptying of the duodenal bulb.
25. The patient's weight should be supported by cushions placed under the thorax and pelvis.
26. to midway between the vertebral column and the lateral border of the abdominal cavity, at the level of L1-L2
27. to the median sagittal plane, at the level of L1-L2
28. Center the film 3 to 6 inches (7.5 to 15 cm) lower.
29. asthenic
30. L1-L2
31. exhalation
32. Have the patient turn toward the left, elevating the left side away from the x-ray table and supporting the raised left side with the left forearm and flexed left knee.
33. 40 to 70
34. hypersthenic
35. on the left side of the abdomen, midway between the vertebral column and the lateral border of the abdomen at the level of L1-L2
36. True
37. False. The patient should suspend respiration after exhalation.
38. supine
39. right
40. 45
41. on the left side of the abdomen, midway between the vertebral column and the lateral border of the abdomen at the level of L1-L2
42. True
43. False. An air-contrast, not barium-filled, image of the pyloric canal and duodenal bulb is produced with the LPO position.
44. A. distal esophagus
    B. fundus
    C. body
    D. pylorus
    E. duodenum
45. a. gas-filled
    b. barium-filled
    c. barium-filled
46. the vertebrae
47. xiphoid process and umbilicus
48. L1-L2
49. L3
50. A. fundus
    B. body
    C. duodenum
    D. duodenal bulb
    E. pyloric portion
51. fundus

52. gas-filled (double-contrast)
53. diaphragmatic herniation (hiatal hernia)
54. a. to midway between the vertebral column and the left lateral border of the abdomen, at the level of L1
    b. to the median sagittal plane, at the level of L1
55. A. fundus
    B. body
    C. pyloric portion
    D. duodenal loop

Exercise 3 The Small Intestine Examination

1. orally, reflux filling, and intubation (direct injection)
2. oral
3. complete reflux filling
4. supine
5. the radiographic procedure by which the small bowel is examined after contrast medium is injected directly into the duodenum by way of a gastric tube that is passed down to the duodenum via the esophagus and stomach
6. duodenum
7. Though instructions may vary, typical preparation may include a restricted diet (soft, low-residue foods) for up to two days before the examination, nothing by mouth after the evening meal the night before the examination, a cleansing enema, and no breakfast on the morning of the examination.
8. enteroclysis, the intubation method
9. to indicate the interval between the exposure of the radiograph and the ingestion of the barium
10. supine
11. 15 minutes
12. 15 to 30 minutes
13. to accelerate peristalsis
14. ileocecal region
15. Entire small intestine should be included on each radiograph.
    Stomach should be included on initial radiographs.
    Time marker should be included.
    Vertebral column should be down the middle of the radiograph.
    Patient should not be rotated.
    Examination is usually completed when barium is visualized in the cecum.
    Exposure factors should penetrate the barium.

Exercise 4 The Large Intestine Examination

1. single-contrast and double-contrast
2. barium sulfate
3. to obtain better coating of the lumen
4. air and carbon dioxide
5. when the patient cannot tolerate retrograde filling of the colon
6. Although it may vary, typical preparation includes a restrictive diet, laxatives, and a cleansing enema.
7. The entire colon should be as clean as possible; no fecal material should be present.

8. approximately 85° to 90° F
9. Barium that is too warm may be unpleasant and debilitating to the patient, may injure internal tissues, and may produce irritation that makes it difficult for the patient to retain the barium for as long as required.
10. approximately 41° F
11. Cold barium causes less irritation to the colon, relaxes the colon, and stimulates tonal contraction of the anal sphincter to aid in increased patient comfort, better toleration of the examination, and improved retention of the barium.
12. Keep the anal sphincter tightly contracted around the enema tip, relax the abdominal muscles, and concentrate on deep oral breathing.
13. 31/2 to 4 inches (8.7 to 10 cm)
14. 18; 24
15. post-evacuation
16. prone
17. iliac crests
18. perpendicularly
19. A. left colic (splenic) flexure
    B. right colic (hepatic) flexure
    C. transverse colon
    D. descending colon
    E. ascending colon
    F. cecum
    G. sigmoid
    H. rectum
20. rectosigmoid
21. 30 to 40 degrees caudad
22. anterior superior iliac spines
23. median sagittal
24. A. left colic (splenic) flexure
    B. transverse colon
    C. sigmoid
    D. rectum
25. False. Superior colic structures (transverse colon and both flexures) need not be demonstrated.
26. True
27. True
28. False. The central ray should be directed perpendicularly to the center of the film.
29. True
30. A. left colic (splenic) flexure
    B. right colic (hepatic) flexure
    C. descending colon
    D. ascending colon
    E. sigmoid
31. left colic (splenic) flexure and descending colon
32. iliac crests
33. A. left colic (splenic) flexure
    B. right colic (hepatic) flexure
    C. transverse colon
    D. descending colon
    E. ascending colon
    F. appendix
    G. sigmoid

34. 2 to 3 inches (5 to 7.5 cm) above the level of the symphysis pubis
35. Hips and femurs should be superimposed.
36. sigmoid; rectum
37. median coronal
38. A. sigmoid
    B. sacrum
    C. rectum
    D. symphysis pubis
39. PA axial
40. cephalically; 30; 40
41. 2 inches (5 cm) below the level of the anterior superior iliac spines
42. the inferior margin of the symphysis pubis
43. A. descending colon
    B. sigmoid
    C. rectum
44. RAO (right PA oblique)
45. 35; 45
46. right
47. right colic (hepatic)
48. A. left colic (splenic) flexure
    B. right colic (hepatic) flexure
    C. descending colon
    D. ascending colon
    E. sigmoid
    F. rectum
49. RPO (right AP oblique)
50. left colic (splenic)
51. 35 to 45
52. A. left colic (splenic) flexure
    B. transverse colon
    C. right colic (hepatic) flexure
    D. descending colon
    E. ascending colon
    F. sigmoid
53. right lateral decubitus
54. Support the patient on a radiolucent pad.
55. a. right lateral decubitus
    b. left lateral decubitus
56. a. Figure 17-20
    b. Figure 17-19
    c. Figure 17-19
    d. Figure 17-20
    e. Figure 17-20
    f. Figure 17-19
57. area from the flexures to the rectum
58. It is lower (generally, 2 to 3 inches [5 to 7.5 cm]), because of the gravitational effect.
59. a. upright
    b. Liquid barium is seen settling to the lower levels of the colon.
60. 1. g
    2. c
    3. e
    4. d

5. a
6. b
7. f
8. h

Self-Test: Anatomy and Positioning of the Alimentary Tract

1. d	14. c	27. d	40. c
2. a	15. a	28. d	41. a
3. c	16. d	29. b	42. c
4. d	17. b	30. b	43. d
5. d	18. d	31. a	44. b
6. b	19. b	32. b	45. c
7. d	20. b	33. c	46. b
8. d	21. a	34. c	47. b
9. b	22. c	35. b	48. b
10. b	23. c	36. a	49. b
11. a	24. d	37. c	50. b
12. d	25. b	38. b	
13. b	26. c	39. b	

Chapter 18: The Urinary System
Part 1: Anatomy of the Urinary System

Exercise 1

1. A. right kidney
   B. inferior vena cava
   C. aorta
   D. left kidney
   E. left ureter
   F. urinary bladder
2. A. left kidney
   B. left ureter
   C. urinary bladder
   D. rectum
   E. prostate
   F. anal canal
3. A. hilum
   B. renal papilla
   C. pelvis
   D. cortical substance
   E. renal sinus
   F. medullary substance
   G. pyramid
   H. minor calyx
   I. major calyx
4. A. cortex
   B. medulla
   C. afferent arteriole
   D. efferent arteriole
   E. glomerulus
   F. distal convoluted tubule

G. glomerular capsule (Bowman's capsule)
H. proximal convoluted tubule
I. descending limb of Henle's loop
J. ascending limb of Henle's loop
K. collecting duct
5. A. ovary
   B. uterine tube
   C. uterus
   D. bladder
   E. pubis
   F. urethra
   G. vagina
   H. rectum
6. A. bladder
   B. pubis
   C. urethra
   D. sacrum
   E. rectum
   F. prostate

Exercise 2

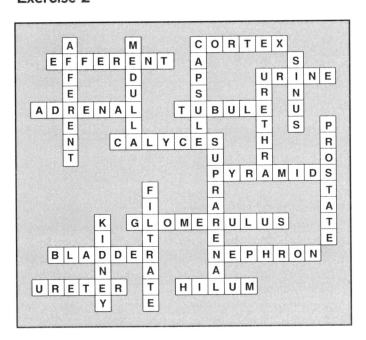

Exercise 3

1. urinary
2. to remove waste material from the blood and excrete it from the body
3. suprarenal (adrenal)
4. hilum
5. medial
6. T12
7. nephron
8. cortex
9. glomerular capsule (Bowman's capsule)
10. glomerulus
11. renal

12. afferent; efferent
13. glomerular filtrate
14. calyces
15. calyces
16. pelvis
17. ureters
18. urinary bladder
19. urethra
20. prostate

Part 2: **Positioning of the Urinary System**

Exercise 1 Excretory Urography

1. urography
2. intravenous urography (IVU) and intravenous pyelography (IVP)
3. iodinated, injectable, ionic or nonionic contrast medium
4. a. warm feeling, flush appearance, urticaria patches, nausea, vomiting, and edema of the respiratory mucous membranes
   b. dyspnea, respiratory arrest, cardiac arrest, renal shutdown, and death
5. within 5 minutes
6. low-residue diet for 1 or 2 days, light evening meal, laxative, and NPO after midnight on the day of the examination
7. to distend the stomach with gas, thus providing a negative background density to better demonstrate renal structures
8. Inappropriate abdominal pressure might retard the excretion of fluid from the kidneys and might cause distortion of ureteral structures.
9. By retarding the flow of opacified urine into the bladder, renal structures are better filled and demonstrated.
10. the anterior surface of the lower abdomen, about 2 inches (5 cm) above the symphysis pubis
11. Rapid releasing of the ureteral compression device might rupture some of the viscera within the pelvis.
12. Increased doses of contrast agents and the use of contrast media of higher concentrations produce better demonstration of ureters.
13. exhalation
14. to demonstrate the mobility of the kidneys
15. patient data, side marker, time-interval, and position indicator
16. to prevent dilution of the opacified urine
17. Elastic waistbands in the underwear can produce unwanted densities in the image because of soft tissue skin folds.
18. to demonstrate the contour of the kidneys; to identify the location of the kidneys; to demonstrate the presence of calculi; to check on how well the patient's gastrointestinal tract was cleaned; and to check the radiographic exposure factors
19. to demonstrate the prostate region
20. to reduce the lordotic curvature and to make the patient more comfortable
21. Tilt the x-ray table and patient to the Trendelenburg position.
22. to obtain a nephrogram

23. 2 to 8 minutes
24. 15; 20
25. Lower the head of the table 15 to 20 degrees Trendelenburg.
26. Make a separate AP projection radiograph of the bladder.
27. 30
28. excessive rotation of the patient
29. bladder
30. A. renal calyces
    B. renal pelvis
    C. abdominal ureter
    D. pelvic ureter
    E. urinary bladder

Exercise 2 Retrograde Urography

1. False. Contrast agents are injected into a selected renal pelvis by means of catheters that pass through the urethra, the bladder, and the ureter to the selected kidney.
2. False. Special cystoscopic-radiographic tables are used for retrograde studies.
3. lithotomy
4. 14 × 17 inches (35 × 43 cm)
5. the urologist
6. The urologist intravenously injects a color dye, and the function of each kidney is determined by the time required for the dye substance to appear in the urine as it passes through the respective catheter.
7. a preliminary radiograph showing catheter insertion, a pyelogram, and a ureterogram
8. By retarding the excretion of the contrast medium from the kidney, the filling of the renal pelvis is enhanced.
9. the ureterogram
10. RPO (right AP oblique) and LPO (left AP oblique)

Exercise 3 Retrograde Cystography

1. by means of a catheter passed through the urethra into the bladder
2. 10 × 12 inches (24 × 30 cm); lengthwise
3. 2 to 3 inches (5 to 7.5 cm) above the upper border of the symphysis pubis
4. to enable the lumbar lordotic curve to arch the pelvis enough to tilt the pubic bones inferiorly
5. perpendicularly, angled 5 degrees caudally, and angled 15 to 20 degrees caudally
6. how much the pelvis is tilted to project the pubic bones inferiorly away from the bladder
7. perpendicularly
8. 2 to 3 inches (5 to 7.5 cm)
9. exhalation
10. lower (distal) ends of the ureters
11. They should be projected below both the bladder and the proximal urethra.
12. 40 to 60
13. perpendicularly and 10 degrees caudally
14. extended and abducted enough to prevent its superimposition on the bladder area

15. a. lateral recumbent
    b. symphysis pubis
    c. perpendicularly

Exercise 4 Male Cystourethrography

1. the radiographic examination of the urinary bladder and urethra after the introduction of a contrast medium by means of a catheter inserted into the bladder
2. A physician inserts a catheter through the urethral canal into the bladder.
3. either RPO (right AP oblique) or LPO (left AP oblique)
4. 35 to 40
5. superior border of the symphysis pubis
6. lengthwise
7. True
8. True
9. False. Only the bladder and urethra need to be demonstrated in their entirety.
10. True

Self-Test: Anatomy and Positioning of the Urinary System

1. a	8. b	15. b	22. b
2. b	9. d	16. c	23. b
3. c	10. b	17. d	24. a
4. b	11. d	18. d	25. b
5. d	12. d	19. d	
6. c	13. a	20. c	
7. c	14. d	21. d	

Chapter 19: Reproductive System
Part 1: Anatomy of the Reproductive Systems

Exercise 1

1. A. uterus
   B. round ligament
   C. ovarian ligament
   D. uterine (fallopian) tube
   E. ovary
2. A. uterine (fallopian) tube
   B. ovary
   C. uterus
   D. round ligament (cut)
   E. urinary bladder
   F. symphysis pubis
   G. urethra
   H. vagina
   I. uterine (fallopian) tube (cut)
   J. cul-de-sac
   K. broad ligament
   L. cervix
   M. uterine ostium (external orifice of cervix)
   N. rectum

3. ovaries
4. ova
5. uterine (fallopian) tube
6. two
7. uterus
8. fundus, body, isthmus, and cervix
9. 1. e
   2. a
   3. b
   4. d
   5. c
10. cervix

Exercise 2

1. A. testicular artery
   B. ductus deferens
   C. rete testis
   D. epididymis
   E. tail of epididymis
   F. head of epididymis
   G. testis
   H. seminiferous tubules
2. A. bladder
   B. pubis
   C. urethra
   D. sacrum
   E. rectum
   F. prostate
3. A. bladder
   B. ductus deferens
   C. ureter
   D. seminal vesicle
   E. ampulla
   F. prostate
   G. epididymis
   H. testis
4. testes (testicles)
5. spermatozoa
6. epididymis
7. ductus deferens
8. ejaculatory
9. prostate
10. urethra

Part 2: Radiography of the Reproductive Systems

Exercise 1 Radiography of the Female Reproductive System

1. hysterosalpingography, pelvic pneumography, and vaginography
2. fetography, pelvimetry, and placentography
3. 1. b
   2. b
   3. d
   4. e

5. c, e, f
6. a, b, d, e
7. a, b
8. f
9. c, f
10. c
11. e
12. f
13. c, e, f
14. f
15. c
4. 1. e
2. d
3. c
4. b
5. a

Exercise 2   Radiography of the Male Reproductive System

1. water-soluble, iodinated
2. to improve radiographic contrast of examined structures
3. prostate
4. prone; because it places the prostate closer to, and the sacrococcygeal vertebrae farther from, the film
5. 20 to 25 degrees cephalad

Self-Test: Reproductive System

1. a	5. b	9. d	13. b
2. b	6. c	10. d	14. c
3. b	7. c	11. d	15. b
4. a	8. a	12. b	

Chapter 20: Skull
Part 1: Osteology of the Skull

Exercise 1

1. A. parietal bone
   B. glabella
   C. greater wing of sphenoid
   D. nasal bone
   E. temporal bone
   F. zygomatic bone
   G. perpendicular plate of ethmoid
   H. vomer
   I. maxilla
   J. frontal bone
   K. sphenoid bone
   L. lacrimal bone
   M. ethmoid bone
   N. middle concha
   O. infraorbital foramen
   P. inferior nasal concha
   Q. anterior nasal spine
   R. mandible

2. A. frontal bone
   B. sphenoid bone
   C. glabella
   D. nasal bone
   E. lacrimal bone
   F. ethmoid bone
   G. anterior nasal spine (acanthion)
   H. zygomatic bone
   I. zygomatic arch
   J. maxilla
   K. mental foramen
   L. mandible
   M. bregma
   N. coronal suture
   O. parietal bone
   P. squamosal suture
   Q. lambda
   R. lambdoidal suture
   S. occipital bone
   T. external occipital protuberance (inion)
   U. mastoid process
   V. temporal bone
   W. external acoustic (auditory) meatus
   X. styloid process

3. A. occipital bone
   B. clivus
   C. petrous portion (pyramid) of temporal bone
   D. temporal bone
   E. foramen spinosum
   F. foramen ovale
   G. chiasmatic (optic) groove or sulcus
   H. greater wing of sphenoid
   I. lesser wing of sphenoid
   J. orbital plate of frontal bone
   K. jugum sphenoidale
   L. crista galli
   M. cribriform plate of ethmoid
   N. optic canal
   O. tuberculum sellae
   P. anterior clinoid process
   Q. sella turcica
   R. posterior clinoid process
   S. foramen lacerum
   T. dorsum sellae
   U. jugular foramen
   V. sigmoid sulcus
   W. basilar portion of occipital bone
   X. hypoglossal canal
   Y. foramen magnum

4. A. frontal bone
   B. frontal sinus
   C. crista galli
   D. nasal bone
   E. ethmoid bone
   F. vomer
   G. maxilla

H. parietal bone
I. sphenoidal sinus
J. petrous portion (pyramid) of temporal bone
K. internal acoustic (auditory) meatus
L. occipital bone
M. squamous portion of temporal bone
N. clivus
O. pterygoid hamulus
P. palatine bone

5. A. squama
   B. frontal eminence (tuberosity)
   C. supraorbital foramen
   D. supraorbital margin
   E. glabella
   F. nasal (frontal) spine
   G. superciliary arch (ridge)
   H. temporal fossa

6. A. perpendicular plate
   B. middle concha
   C. crista galli
   D. air cells of labyrinth
   E. cribriform plate

7. A. occipital angle
   B. mastoid angle
   C. superior sagittal suture
   D. frontal angle
   E. sphenoid angle

8. A. pterygoid hamulus
   B. lateral pterygoid lamina
   C. dorsum sellae
   D. posterior clinoid processes
   E. anterior clinoid processes
   F. optic canal
   G. lesser wing
   H. superior orbital fissure
   I. greater wing

9. A. squama
   B. foramen magnum
   C. basilar part
   D. condyle
   E. external occipital protuberance (inion)

10. A. squama
    B. mastoid portion
    C. external acoustic (auditory) meatus
    D. tympanic portion
    E. styloid process
    F. mandibular fossa
    G. articular tubercle
    H. zygomatic process
    I. petrous portion

11. A. external acoustic (auditory) meatus
    B. cartilage
    C. tympanic membrane
    D. auditory ossicles
    E. semicircular canals
    F. stapes (in oval window)

G. internal acoustic (auditory) meatus
H. cochlear nerve
I. cochlea
J. round window
K. tensor tympani muscle
L. auditory (eustachian) tube
M. nasopharynx
N. anterior (supratragal) notch
O. infraorbitomeatal line
P. intertragal (infratragal) notch

12. A. neck
    B. condyle
    C. alveolar process
    D. mental foramen
    E. symphysis
    F. coronoid process
    G. ramus
    H. body
    I. mental protuberance
    J. angle
    K. gonion

13. A. body
    B. greater cornu
    C. lesser cornu

Exercise 2

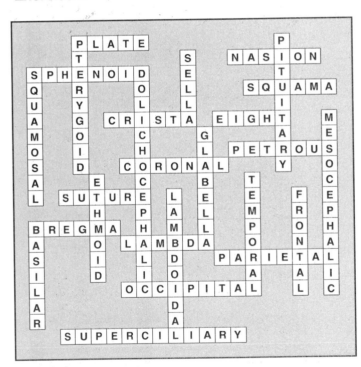

Exercise 3

1. a
2. a
3. c
4. d
5. d

6. f
7. b
8. d
9. f
10. b
11. e
12. f
13. e
14. d
15. e
16. a
17. b
18. d
19. d
20. d

Exercise 4

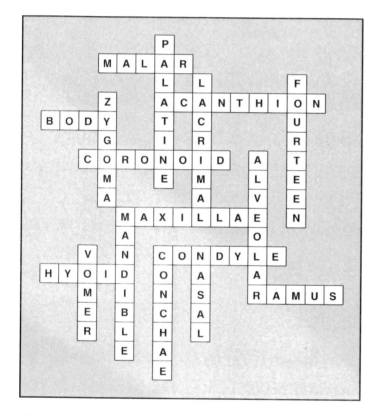

Exercise 5

1. cranial; facial
2. frontal, 1; ethmoid, 1; parietal, 2; sphenoid, 1; temporal, 2; and occipital, 1
3. nasal, 2; lacrimal, 2; maxillae, 2; zygomatic, 2; palatine, 2; inferior nasal conchae, 2; vomer, 1; and mandible, 1
4. flat
5. diploë
6. bregma and lambda
7. bregma
8. lambda
9. mesocephalic, 47; brachycephalic, 54; and dolichocephalic, 40

10. frontal
11. ethmoid
12. parietals
13. tuber (tuberosity or eminence)
14. sagittal
15. coronal
16. occipital
17. lambdoidal
18. sphenoid
19. occipital
20. basilar
21. foramen magnum
22. sphenoid
23. C1 vertebra (atlas)
24. sphenoid
25. temporal
26. tympanic
27. mastoid
28. petrous portion (pars petrosa; petrous pyramid)
29. temporal
30. auricle (pinna)
31. malleus (hammer), incus (anvil), and stapes (stirrup)
32. temporal
33. temporal
34. nasal
35. lacrimal
36. maxilla
37. antrum of Highmore
38. alveolar process
39. maxillae
40. acanthion
41. zygomatic
42. zygoma and malar
43. palatine
44. inferior nasal conchae
45. vomer
46. mandible
47. ramus
48. hyoid
49. condyle and coronoid process
50. condyle

Part 2: **Radiography of the Skull**

Exercise 1 **Skull Topography**

1. A. angle of mandible (gonion)
   B. infraorbitomeatal margin
   C. outer canthus
   D. median sagittal plane
   E. glabella
   F. interpupillary line
   G. inner canthus
   H. nasion
   I. acanthion
   J. mental point
2. A. auricular point

B. angle of mandible (gonion)
C. glabellomeatal line
D. orbitomeatal line
E. infraorbitomeatal line
F. acanthomeatal line
G. glabelloalveolar line
H. glabella
I. nasion
J. acanthion
K. mental point

3. a. posterior surface of the occipital bone
   b. superior aspect of the cranium where the parietal bones join together
   c. angle of the mandible; lateroposterior aspect of the mandible
   d. midpoint of the frontonasal suture
   e. smooth elevation between the superciliary ridges
   f. midpoint of the anterior nasal spine
   g. midpoint of the mental protuberance; anterior aspect of the mandible where the two mandibular bodies join together
   h. lateral aspect of each orbit where the two eyelids originate
   i. raised prominence just above each orbit on the frontal bone; coincides with the eyebrows

4. a. interpupillary line
   b. orbitomeatal line
   c. glabellomeatal line
   d. infraorbitomeatal line
   e. acanthomeatal line
   f. glabelloalveolar line
   g. orbitomeatal line
   h. infraorbitomeatal line
   i. median sagittal plane

5. a. 7
   b. 8

Exercise 2 Positioning for the Cranium

1. a. parallel
   b. perpendicular
2. infraorbitomeatal line
3. 2 inches (5 cm) above the external acoustic meatus
4. 10 X 12 inches (24 X 30 cm); crosswise
5. perpendicular to a point approximately 2 inches (5 cm) above the external acoustic meatus
6. Elevate the head on a radiolucent sponge.
7. False. The central ray should enter at a point 2 inches (5 cm) superior to the external acoustic meatus.
8. False. The TMJ closer to the film is seen in better recorded detail than is the TMJ remote from the film.
9. Entire cranium should be demonstrated without rotation or tilt.
   Mandibular rami should be superimposed.
   Orbital roofs should be superimposed.
   Mastoid regions should be superimposed.
   External acoustic meatuses should be superimposed.
   Temporomandibular joints should be superimposed.

Sella turcica should not be rotated.
Parietal region should be penetrated.
Mandible should not overlap cervical vertebrae.

10. a. A support should be placed under the thorax to raise the inferior aspect of the head and to place the median sagittal plane parallel with the film.
    b. A radiolucent sponge should be placed under the head to make the median sagittal plane parallel with the film.

11. a. Figure 20-19. Certain structures of the skull are superimposed with their opposite side (orbital roofs, mandibular rami, mastoid regions, external acoustic meatuses, and temporomandibular joints), and no rotation is seen.
    b. Figure 20-18. Cranial structures (orbital roofs, temporomandibular joints, and external acoustic meatuses) are longitudinally separated.
    c. Figure 20-17. Cranial structures (orbital roofs, temporomandibular joints, and external acoustic meatuses) are laterally separated.
    d. Figure 20-18

12. A. posterior clinoid process
    B. orbital roof
    C. anterior clinoid process
    D. sella turcica (hypophyseal fossa)
    E. dorsum sellae
    F. temporomandibular joint
    G. mastoid region
    H. mandibular rami

13. a. perpendicular
    b. perpendicular
14. forehead and nose
15. a. perpendicular
    b. 15 degrees caudad
    c. 20 to 25 degrees caudad
    d. 25 to 30 degrees caudad
16. nasion
17. nasion
18. Stop breathing.
19. Distance from the lateral border of the skull to the lateral border of the orbit should be equal on both sides.
    Petrous ridges should be symmetric.
    Petrous bones should lie in the lower one-third of the orbit, with a central ray angulation of 15 degrees caudad, and should fill the orbits with no central ray angulation.
    Frontal bone should be penetrated without excessive density at the lateral borders of the skull.
    Entire cranial vertex should be included.
20. a. caudally 15 degrees; petrous ridges lie in the lower one-third of the orbits
    b. perpendicularly; petrous ridges fill the orbits
21. a. caudally 15 degrees
    b. lower one-third of the orbits
    c. The distance from the lateral border of the skull to the lateral border of the orbit is not equal on both sides.
    d. The head is rotated, moving the occipital bone closer to the left shoulder; the median sagittal plane is not perpendicular to the film.

22. a. perpendicular to the nasion
    b. Petrous ridges should fill the orbits.
    c. yes
    d. The distance from the lateral border of the skull to the lateral border of the orbit is not equal on both sides.
    e. The head is rotated, moving the occipital bone closer to the right shoulder; the median sagittal plane is not perpendicular to the film.
23. a. acceptable
    b. unacceptable
    c. The head is rotated, moving the occipital bone closer to the left shoulder; the median sagittal plane is not perpendicular to the film.
    d. perpendicularly
24. A. dorsum sellae
    B. superior orbital shadow (margin)
    C. sphenoid plane
    D. petrous ridge
    E. ethmoidal sinus
    F. inferior orbital shadow (margin)
    G. crista galli
25. Towne
26. highest point of the vertex
27. orbitomeatal; infraorbitomeatal
28. 30 degrees caudad and 37 degrees caudad; 2 to 2 1/2 inches (5 to 6.25 cm) above the glabella
29. the positioning line (orbitomeatal or infraorbitomeatal) that is perpendicular to the film
30. Distance from the lateral border of the skull to the lateral border of the foramen magnum should be equal on both sides.
    Petrous pyramids should be symmetric.
    Dorsum sellae and posterior clinoid processes should be visualized within the foramen magnum.
    Occipital bone should be penetrated without excessive density at the lateral borders of the skull.
31. A. parietal bone
    B. occipital bone
    C. foramen magnum
    D. petrous ridge
    E. posterior clinoid process
    F. dorsum sellae
32. True
33. False. Hypersthenic patients must be either prone or upright.
34. False. The PA axial projection (Haas method) is sometimes referred to as the reverse Towne method.
35. orbitomeatal
36. **25 degrees cephalad**
37. **on the median sagittal** plane at a point approximately 1 1/2 **inches (3.7 cm) below** the external occipital protuberance **(inion)**
38. **Dorsum sellae should** be seen and projected within the **foramen magnum.**
    Distance from the lateral border of the skull to the lateral border of the foramen magnum should be equal on both sides.

Petrous pyramids should be symmetric.
Entire cranium should be included.
39. A. occipital bone
    B. foramen magnum
    C. petrous ridge
    D. posterior clinoid process
    E. dorsum sellae
40. a. perpendicular
    b. parallel
41. infraorbitomeatal
42. on the median sagittal plane of the throat between the angles of the mandible and passing through a point 3/4 inch (1.9 cm) anterior to the level of the external acoustic meatus
43. Distance from the lateral border of the skull to the mandibular condyles should be equal on both sides.
    Mandibular symphysis should superimpose anterior frontal bone.
    Mandibular condyles should be anterior to the petrous pyramids.
    Petrosae should be symmetric.
    Structures of the cranial base should be clearly visible as indicated by adequate penetration.
44. Mandibular symphysis does not superimpose the anterior frontal bone.
45. A. maxillary sinus
    B. ethmoidal air cells
    C. mandible
    D. vomer
    E. sphenoidal sinus
    F. clivus
    G. foramen spinosum
    H. mandibular condyle
    I. dens (odontoid process)
    J. petrosa
    K. mastoid process

Exercise 3 Positioning for the Sella Turcica

1. a. parallel
   b. perpendicular
   c. parallel
2. at a point 3/4 inch (1.9 cm) anterior to and 3/4 inch (1.9 cm) superior to the external acoustic meatus
3. Stop breathing.
4. Sella turcica should not be rotated.
   Anterior clinoid processes should be superimposed.
   Posterior clinoid processes should be superimposed.
   Sella turcica should be in the center of the radiograph.
5. A. anterior clinoid process
   B. posterior clinoid process
   C. dorsum sellae
   D. hypophyseal (pituitary) fossa
   E. sphenoidal sinus

Exercise 4 Positioning for the Optic Canal (Foramen)

1. zygomatic bone (cheek area), nose, and chin
2. acanthomeatal line
3. 53
4. True
5. True
6. True
7. False. Incorrect angulation of the acanthomeatal line causes longitudinal deviation from the preferred location of the optic canal. (Any lateral deviation of the preferred location for the optic canal is caused by incorrect rotation of the head.)
8. False. The central ray should be directed perpendicularly through the affected orbit closer to the film.
9. a. Figure 20-33. The optic canal is demonstrated in the inferior and lateral quadrant of the orbit.
   b. Figure 20-32. The position of the optic canal is posterior to the lateral orbital margin.
   c. Figure 20-34. The position of the optic canal is too much toward the medial aspect of the orbit.
10. A. superior orbital margin
    B. lateral orbital margin
    C. optic canal
    D. medial orbital margin
    E. lesser wing of sphenoid
    F. ethmoidal sinus
    G. inferior orbital margin
11. parieto-orbital oblique
12. supine
13. True
14. False. The orbitoparietal oblique projection results in a greater amount of radiation exposure to the lens of the eye than does the parieto-orbital oblique projection.
15. False. The orbitoparietal oblique projection is the AP oblique projection for the orbit. (The PA oblique projection for the orbit is the parieto-orbital oblique projection.)
16. True
17. acanthomeatal line
18. median sagittal
19. a. The position of the optic canal is laterally deviated from the preferred location.
    b. The angle formed by the median sagittal plane and the film was less than the required 53 degrees.
    c. Rotate the head, moving the occipital bone away from the film until the median sagittal plane forms an angle of 53 degrees with the film.
20. Optic canal should lie in the inferior and lateral quadrant of the orbit.
    Optic canal should be seen enface at the end of the sphenoid ridge.
    Entire orbital shadow should be included.
    Close beam restriction of the orbital region is needed.

Chapter 21: **Facial Bones**

Radiography of the Facial Bones

Exercise 1 Positioning for Facial Bones and Nasal Bones

1. median sagittal
2. interpupillary
3. infraorbitomeatal
4. zygomatic
5. to prevent rotation
6. lateral surface of the zygomatic bone
7. All facial bones should be completely included with the zygomatic bone in the center.
   Mandibular rami should be almost perfectly superimposed.
   Orbital roofs should be superimposed.
   Sella turcica should not be rotated.
8. The mandibular rami are not superimposed, and the orbital roofs are not superimposed.
9. A. frontal sinus
   B. nasal bone
   C. sella turcica
   D. maxillary sinus
   E. external acoustic (auditory) meatus
   F. maxilla
   G. mandible
10. a. 37-degree angulation
    b. perpendicular
11. acanthion
12. Distance between the lateral border of the skull and orbit should be equal on both sides.
    Petrous ridges should be projected immediately below the maxillae.
13. a. Petrous ridges will be projected too far below maxillae, and maxillae will appear foreshortened.
    b. Petrous ridges will superimpose maxillary sinuses.
14. a. Figure 21-5
    b. Figure 21-3
    c. Figure 21-4
15. A. orbit
    B. zygomatic arch
    C. maxillary sinus
    D. maxilla
    E. petrous ridge
    F. mandibular angle
16. supine
17. parietoacanthial; Waters
18. median sagittal plane and infraorbitomeatal line
19. approximately 3 inches (7.5 cm) above the external occipital protuberance
20. Stop breathing.
21. 30 degrees cephalad
22. lips

23. **Distance between** the lateral border of the skull and orbit **should be equal** on both sides.

    Petrous ridges should be projected in the maxillary sinuses.

24. A. orbit

    B. zygomatic bone

    C. maxillary sinus

    D. petrous ridge

25. a. perpendicular

    b. parallel

26. two

27. nasion

28. perpendicular to the bridge of the nose at a point 3/4 inch (1.9 cm) distal to the nasion

29. Nasal bone and soft tissue should be demonstrated without rotation.

    Anterior nasal spine and frontonasal suture should be visualized.

30. A. frontonasal (nasofrontal) suture

    B. nasal bone

    C. anterior nasal spine of maxilla

Exercise 2 Positioning for Zygomatic Arches

1. True

2. False. Zygomatic arches should be free from overlying structures.

3. False. The posterior cranium need not be included in the image.

4. False. The median sagittal plane should be perpendicular to the film.

5. infraorbitomeatal

6. submentovertical

7. perpendicular to the infraorbitomeatal line and centered on the median sagittal plane midway between the zygomatic arches, passing through a coronal plane approximately 1 inch (2.5 cm) posterior to the outer canthus

8. Zygomatic arches should be free from overlying structures.

    Zygomatic arches should be symmetric and without foreshortening.

    There should be no rotation of the head.

9. a. Zygomatic arches are not symmetric, and the left zygomatic arch is superimposed with cranial structures.

    b. The median sagittal plane was not perpendicular to the film because the patient's head was slightly tilted.

10. False. Zygomatic arches are demonstrated individually with the tangential projection.

11. True

12. infraorbitomeatal

13. perpendicularly to the infraorbitomeatal line and centered to the zygomatic arch

14. Zygomatic arch should be free from overlying structures.

15. a. perpendicular

    b. perpendicular

16. a. 30 degrees caudad

    b. 37 degrees caudad

17. nasion

18. True

19. False. Close beam restriction to zygomatic arches and adjacent structures may exclude the vertex.

20. A. occipital bone

    B. mandible

    C. zygomatic arch

Exercise 3 Positioning for the Mandible

1. forehead and nose

2. tip of the nose

3. perpendicular

4. Stop breathing for the exposure.

5. acanthion

6. True

7. False. The central portion of the mandible is superimposed with the cervical vertebrae.

8. Mandibular body and rami should be symmetric on both sides.

    Entire mandible should be included.

9. a. Base of the occipital partially superimposes the mandible, and the mandibular rami are not seen without superimposition from surrounding structures.

    b. Reposition the head, ensuring that the forehead is in contact with the vertical grid device or x-ray table surface, to image the mandible without cranial superimposition.

10. A. condyle

    B. mastoid process

    C. fracture of the mandibular ramus

    D. body

11. forehead and nose

12. glabella

13. perpendicular

14. Stop breathing for the exposure.

15. 20 to 25 degrees cephalad

16. superimposition with the spine

17. Mandibular body and rami should be symmetric on both sides.

    Condylar processes should be clearly demonstrated.

    Entire mandible should be demonstrated.

18. False. The head is rotated from true lateral so that the broad surface of the mandibular surface is parallel with the film.

19. False. The central ray should be directed 25 degrees cephalad.

20. body

21. slightly posterior to the mandibular angle on the side farther from the film

22. From true lateral rotate the head, moving the face closer to the film, until the broad surface of the mandibular body is parallel with the film.

23. body

24. Mandibular body to canine tooth should be demonstrated.

    Opposite side of the mandible should not overlap mandibular body.

25. a. Opposite side of the mandible superimposes the mandibular body.
    b. Position the head so that the uppermost side of the mandible will be projected above the mandibular body closer to the film.
26. A. coronoid process
    B. condyle
    C. ramus
    D. body
    E. angle (gonion)
27. True
28. False. The head should be slightly rotated from a lateral position to place the broad surface of the mandibular body parallel with the film.
29. False. The view of the axiolateral oblique projection does not show the center part of the mandibular body superimposed with the spine.
30. True
31. True
32. 20 degrees cephalad
33. approximately 2 inches (5 cm) distal to the mandibular angle on the side farther from the film
34. Stop breathing for the exposure.
35. a. side of chin
    b. cheek

Exercise 4 Positioning for the Temporomandibular Joints

1. True
2. False. The head should be placed in the AP position.
3. Occlusion of the incisors places the mandible in a position of protrusion in which the condyles are carried out of the mandibular fossae.
4. any trauma to the mandible where the mandible is suspected to be fractured; because of the danger of fracture displacement
5. median sagittal plane and orbitomeatal line
6. directly below the TMJs
7. 35 degrees caudad
8. on the median sagittal plane at a point 3 inches (7.5 cm) above the nasion
9. The head should not be rotated.
   There should be only minimal superimposition by the petrosa on the condyle.
10. The head should not be rotated.
    Condyle and temporomandibular articulation should be demonstrated below the petrosa.
11. The median sagittal plane should form a 15-degree angle with the film.
12. acanthomeatal
13. 1/2 inch (1.2 cm) anterior to the external acoustic (auditory) meatus
14. 15 degrees caudad
15. False. In order to exit through the external acoustic (auditory) meatus closer to the film, the caudally directed

central ray should enter slightly posterior and superior to the uppermost external acoustic (auditory) meatus.
16. True
17. False. Close beam restriction should surround the affected TMJ.
18. in the mandibular fossa
19. the TMJ closer to the film
20. A. mandibular fossa
    B. articular tubercle
    C. condyle

Chapter 22: **Paranasal Sinuses**

Chapter 22 Review

1. frontal, sphenoidal, ethmoidal, and maxillary
2. A. sphenoidal sinuses
   B. maxillary sinuses
   C. frontal sinuses
   D. ethmoidal sinuses (air cells)
3. frontal
4. maxillary
5. sphenoidal
6. sphenoidal
7. anterior; middle; posterior
8. upright (erect)
9. to demonstrate the presence or absence of fluid and to differentiate between shadows caused by fluid and those caused by other pathologic conditions
10. Underpenetration produces shadows simulating pathologic conditions that do not exist.
11. median sagittal; parallel
12. interpupillary; perpendicular
13. a point 1/2 to 1 inch (1.2 to 2.5 cm) posterior to the adjacent outer canthus
14. sphenoidal
15. all four
16. All four sinus groups should be included.
    Sella turcica should not be rotated.
    Orbital roof should be superimposed.
    Mandibular rami should be superimposed.
    Sinuses should be visualized clearly.
    Close beam restriction of the sinus area is needed.
17. A. frontal sinus
    B. hypophyseal fossa
    C. sphenoidal sinus
    D. ethmoidal air cells
    E. maxillary sinus
    F. superimposed mandibular rami
18. a. glabellomeatal
    b. orbitomeatal
19. a. 23 degrees caudad
    b. 15 degrees caudad
20. angled 15 degrees, open posteroinferiorly (tilt the top of the grid device toward the patient)
21. nasion

22. frontal; anterior ethmoidal
23. in the lower one-third of the orbits
24. Distance between the lateral border of the skull and the lateral border of the orbits should be equal.
   Petrous ridges should be symmetric on both sides.
   Petrous ridges should lie in the lower one-third of the orbits.
   Frontal sinuses should lie above the frontonasal suture and anterior ethmoidal air cells above the petrous ridges.
   Frontal and anterior ethmoidal sinuses should be visualized clearly.
   Close beam restriction of the sinus area is needed.
25. A. frontal sinus
   B. frontonasal suture
   C. ethmoidal air cells
   D. petrous ridge
   E. sphenoidal air cells
   F. maxillary sinus
26. maxillary
27. sphenoidal
28. immediately below maxillary sinuses
29. superimposed with maxillary sinuses
30. foreshortened
31. False. Only the chin should touch the vertical grid device.
32. True
33. orbitomeatal
34. acanthion
35. sphenoidal
36. Petrous pyramids should lie immediately inferior to the floor of the maxillary sinuses.
   Distance from the lateral border of the skull to the lateral border of the orbit should be equal on both sides.
   Orbits and maxillary sinuses should be symmetric on both sides.
   Maxillary sinuses should be visualized clearly.
   Close beam restriction of the sinus area is needed.
   Sphenoidal sinuses are seen projected through the open mouth if modification is performed.
37. A. frontal sinus
   B. ethmoidal air cells
   C. foramen rotundum
   D. maxillary sinus
   E. petrous pyramid
   F. mastoid air cells
38. True
39. False. The infraorbitomeatal line should be as nearly parallel with the film as possible.
40. True
41. True
42. True
43. False. To demonstrate paranasal sinuses, close restriction of the beam to the sinus area may exclude the occipital bone.
44. Distance from the lateral border of the skull to the mandibular condyle will not be equal on both sides.
45. sphenoidal and ethmoidal

46. Mandibular symphysis should superimpose anterior frontal bone.
47. The infraorbitomeatal line was not parallel with the film because the neck was not extended enough (assuming the central ray was correctly directed).
48. The infraorbitomeatal line was not parallel with the film because the neck was extended too far or the vertical cassette holder was tilted too far toward the patient (assuming the central ray was correctly directed).
49. anterior to the petrous ridges
50. A. maxillary sinus
   B. ethmoidal sinus
   C. mandible
   D. vomer
   E. sphenoidal sinus
   F. clivus
   G. foramen spinosum
   H. mandibular condyle
   I. dens (odontoid process)
   J. petrosa
   K. mastoid process
51. True
52. True
53. False. Close beam restriction should be limited to the sinus area.
54. False. Respiration should be suspended for the exposure.
55. orbitomeatal
56. a. perpendicular to the nasion
   b. 10 degrees cephalad to the glabella
   c. perpendicular to midway between the infraorbital margins and acanthion
57. superior to the anterior ethmoidal air cells
58. through the frontal bone, superior to the frontal sinuses
59. inferior to the base of the cranium
60. Distance between the lateral border of the skull and the median sagittal plane should be equal on both sides.
   Petrous pyramids should be symmetric on both sides.
   Close beam restriction of the sinus area is needed.

Chapter 23: **Temporal Bone**

Chapter 23 Review

1. False. The head should be rotated 15 degrees from true lateral, moving the face closer to the film.
2. False. The head should be rotated 15 degrees from true lateral, moving the face closer to the film.
3. True
4. From true lateral with the affected mastoid centered to the film, rotate the head until the median sagittal plane forms a 15-degree angle with the film.
5. Tape the auricle of the ear forward.
6. right side; closer to
7. to a point 1 inch (2.5 cm) posterior to the external acoustic meatus of the side adjacent to the film
8. 15 degrees caudad

9. approximately 2 inches (5 cm) posterior and 2 inches (5 cm) above the uppermost external acoustic meatus

10. Mastoid closer to the film should be included, with the air cells demonstrated and centered to the film.
Opposite mastoid should not superimpose but should lie inferior and slightly anterior to the mastoid of interest.
Auricle of the ear should not superimpose the mastoid.
Internal and external acoustic meatus should be superimposed.
Temporomandibular joint should be visualized anterior to the mastoid.
Close beam restriction of the mastoid region is needed.

11. A. tegmen tympani
B. internal and external acoustic meatus
C. mastoid air cells
D. sigmoid sinus sulcus
E. mastoid process
F. mandibular condyle

12. on each cheek at a point 1 inch (2.5 cm) anterior to the external acoustic meatus

13. forehead, nose, and zygomatic bone (zygoma)

14. 53

15. infraorbitomeatal

16. 12 degrees cephalad

17. right side; closer to

18. A. occipital bone
B. internal acoustic canal
C. arcuate eminence
D. mastoid air cells
E. external acoustic meatus and canal
F. mandibular condyle
G. mastoid process

19. False. The median sagittal plane should form an angle of 53 degrees with the film.

20. True

21. True

22. right side; farther from

23. 10 degrees caudad

24. on the zygomatic bone approximately 1 inch (2.5 cm) anterior to and 3/4 inch (1.9 cm) above the external acoustic meatus

25. Petrosa and petrous ridge should be demonstrated in profile.
Lateral border of the skull to lateral border of the orbit should be included.
Petrous ridge should lie horizontally and at a point approximately two-thirds of the way up the lateral border of the orbit.
Mastoid should be demonstrated in profile below the margin of the cranium.
Posterior surface of the ramus should parallel lateral surface of the cervical vertebrae.
Mandibular condyle will be projected over the first cervical vertebra near the petrosa.

Chapter 24: **Mammography**
Part 1: **Anatomy and Physiology of the Breast**

1. A. axillary prolongation (tail) of breast
B. serratus anterior
C. pectoralis minor
D. pectoralis major (cut)

2. A. fat
B. nipple
C. lactiferous tubules
D. fat
E. inframammary crease
F. pectoralis major
G. retromammary fat

3. to produce and secrete milk

4. mammary

5. areola

6. 15; 20

7. acini

8. Lobules decrease in size as the patient ages.

9. the normal process of changes in breast tissues (lobules decrease in size, and glandular and parenchymal tissues are replaced by fat) that occur as the patient ages

10. fat

11. to drain milk from lobes

12. tail

13. Cooper's

14. axilla

15. sternum

Part 2: **Radiography of the Breast**

1. film-screen and xeromammography

2. film-screen; less radiation exposure to the patient, faster processing time, and ability to produce more detailed images

3. film-screen

4. 1

5. 22 to 28 kVp

6. 55 kVp

7. tungsten

8. molybdenum

9. tungsten

10. Tungsten targets are unable to produce the low-energy x-ray photons that are ideally suited for mammography.

11. 0.3 (units used for magnification studies have focal spots as small as 0.1 mm)

12. close to and aligned with the chest wall

13. 24; 60

14. to produce more uniform breast thickness

15. As the maximum thickness of the breast is decreased by compression, the exposure time is reduced.

16. Compression produces a radiograph of more uniform density.

17. Compression pushes all the contents of the breast closer to the x-ray film, further decreasing geometric distortion.

18. Chest wall is not well visualized.
19. Cloth produces artifacts in mammographic images.
20. craniocaudal and mediolateral oblique
21. directed straightforward and in profile
22. along the lateral side
23. mediolateral oblique
24. standing or sitting, facing the film holder
25. four

Self-Test: Mammography

1. a		6. d	
2. a		7. b	
3. d		8. c	
4. c		9. c	
5. b		10. d	

Chapter 25: **Central Nervous System**
Part 1: **Anatomy of the Central Nervous System**

1. A. cerebrum
   B. corpus callosum
   C. cerebrum
   D. cerebellum
   E. hypophysis cerebri (pituitary gland)
   F. medulla oblongata
   G. cerebellum
   H. pons
2. A. gray substance
   B. white substance
   C. posterior nerve root
   D. anterior nerve root
3. A. pons
   B. medulla oblongata
   C. spinal cord
   D. dural sac for cauda equina
4. A. fourth ventricle
   B. inferior horn
   C. interventricular foramen
   D. anterior horn
   E. body of lateral ventricle
   F. third ventricle
   G. posterior horn
   H. cerebral aqueduct
5. A. body of lateral ventricle
   B. anterior horn
   C. inferior horn
6. A. fourth ventricle
   B. body of lateral ventricle
   C. third ventricle
   D. anterior horn
   E. inferior horn
   F. lateral recess
   G. posterior horn

7. brain and spinal cord
8. cerebrum, cerebellum, and brain stem
9. diencephalon, midbrain (mesencephalon), pons, and medulla oblongata
10. cerebellum, pons, and medulla oblongata
11. cerebrum (forebrain)
12. forebrain
13. midbrain (mesencephalon)
14. longitudinal fissure
15. pituitary gland
16. cerebellum
17. medulla oblongata
18. meninges
19. pia mater
20. dura mater
21. lateral
22. cerebrum (forebrain)
23. interventricular
24. foramen of Monro
25. cerebral aqueduct and aqueduct of Sylvius

Part 2: **Radiography of the Central Nervous System**

1. radiographic examination of the spinal cord after the injection of a contrast medium into the subarachnoid space
2. L2-L3, L3-L4, and cisterna cerebellomedullaris (cisterna magna)
3. extrinsic spinal cord compression
4. nonionic, water-soluble; they provide good visualization of nerve roots and good enhancement for follow-up CT and are readily absorbed by the body
5. to prevent it from accidentally contacting the spinal needle
6. Explain details of the examination to the patient before beginning the procedure.
7. prone and lateral recumbent with the spine flexed
8. varying the angulation of the table
9. to compress the cisterna cerebellomedullaris and thus prevent the contrast medium from entering cranial structures
10. cross-table lateral of the cervical spine

Self-Test: Central Nervous System

1. b		6. b		11. a	
2. b		7. c		12. b	
3. c		8. d		13. a	
4. b		9. c		14. c	
5. b		10. d		15. c	

Chapter 26: **Circulatory System**
Part 1: **Anatomy of the Circulatory System**

Exercise 1

1. A. superior sagittal sinus
   B. transverse sinus
   C. internal jugular vein
   D. right subclavian artery and vein
   E. superior vena cava
   F. brachial artery and basilic vein
   G. celiac axis (artery)
   H. portal vein
   I. renal artery and vein
   J. superior mesenteric artery and vein
   K. common iliac artery and vein
   L. common femoral artery and vein
   M. popliteal artery
   N. anterior tibial artery
   O. posterior tibial artery
   P. anterior facial artery and vein
   Q. common carotid artery
   R. aortic arch
   S. pulmonary artery and vein
   T. aorta
   U. inferior vena cava
   V. inferior mesenteric vein
   W. radial artery and cephalic vein
   X. ulnar artery and basilic vein
   Y. deep femoral artery
   Z. superficial femoral artery
   AA. popliteal vein
   BB. large saphenous vein
2. A. aortic arch
   B. superior vena cava
   C. right pulmonary artery
   D. right pulmonary veins
   E. right atrium
   F. right atrioventricular (tricuspid) valve
   G. right ventricle
   H. inferior vena cava
   I. descending aorta
   J. left ventricle
   K. left atrioventricular (bicuspid or mitral) valve
   L. left lung
   M. left atrium
3. A. right coronary artery
   B. left coronary artery
4. A. coronary sinus
   B. great cardiac vein
5. A. capillaries
   B. lungs
   C. right atrium
   D. right ventricle
   E. liver
   F. intestine

G. aorta
H. left atrium
I. left ventricle
J. stomach
K. spleen
L. pancreas

6. A. external carotid artery
   B. internal carotid artery
   C. right common carotid artery
   D. right vertebral artery
   E. right subclavian artery
   F. brachiocephalic artery
   G. brachial artery
   H. radial artery
   I. ulnar artery
   J. left subclavian artery
   K. left vertebral artery
   L. left common carotid artery
   M. thyroid
7. A. axillary nodes
   B. common iliac nodes
   C. deep inguinal nodes
   D. cervical nodes
   E. thoracic duct
   F. lumbar nodes
   G. superior inguinal nodes

Exercise 2

1. blood-vascular; lymphatic
2. pulmonary; systemic
3. pulmonary
4. arteries
5. veins
6. arterioles
7. capillaries
8. venules
9. venules
10. pulmonary
11. superior vena cava
12. inferior vena cava
13. myocardium
14. endocardium
15. epicardium
16. left ventricle; because the left ventricle pumps blood through the systemic circulation system
17. between the two walls of the pericardial sac
18. atria
19. ventricles
20. atria
21. ventricles
22. tricuspid
23. mitral valve and bicuspid valve
24. right
25. left
26. left ventricle
27. coronary

28. cardiac
29. right
30. aorta
31. iliac
32. femoral
33. popliteal
34. tibial
35. portal
36. hepatic
37. inferior vena cava
38. pulmonary
39. pulmonary
40. pulmonary
41. systole
42. diastole
43. right and left common carotid arteries and right and left vertebral arteries
44. left common carotid artery
45. subclavian
46. basilar
47. internal; external
48. cerebral
49. posterior cerebral
50. jugular
51. brachiocephalic
52. subclavian
53. brachial
54. radial; ulnar
55. forearm
56. aorta (abdominal)
57. brain
58. heart
59. thoracic duct
60. subclavian; jugular

Part 2: **Radiography of the Circulatory System**

1. There is reduced risk of extravasation; most body parts can be reached for selective injection; the patient can be positioned as needed; and the catheter can be safely left in the body while the radiographs are being examined.
2. Seldinger
3. femoral
4. to stabilize the catheter tip by reducing whiplash during injection of the contrast medium
5. sweating and nausea caused by a drop in blood pressure
6. The patient's legs should be elevated and intravenous fluids may be administered.
7. shallow breathing, high pulse rate, and loss of consciousness
8. to reduce the possibility of aspiration of vomitus
9. to saturate the kidneys and minimize kidney damage from iodinated contrast media
10. T6
11. A. brachiocephalic artery
   B. ascending aorta
   C. right coronary artery
   D. intercostal arteries
   E. left common carotid artery
   F. left subclavian artery
   G. left coronary artery
   H. descending thoracic aorta
12. from the diaphragm to the aortic bifurcation
13. lateral
14. A. hepatic artery
   B. right renal artery
   C. right common iliac artery
   D. splenic artery
   E. left renal artery
   F. abdominal aorta
15. A. celiac axis
   B. superior mesenteric artery
   C. abdominal aorta
16. AP
17. expiration
18. A. left gastric artery
   B. hepatic artery
   C. gastroduodenal artery
   D. splenic artery
   E. celiac axis
19. to ensure exact positioning of the tube-part-film alignment and close collimation of the x-ray tube
20. splenic
21. proximally
22. upper
23. subclavian
24. common iliac
25. subclavian
26. A. ulnar artery
   B. posterior interosseous artery
   C. brachial artery
   D. right subclavian artery
27. superficial vein at the wrist (for demonstrating the entire upper limb) or at the elbow (for demonstrating the upper arm)
28. A. cephalic vein
   B. basilic vein
   C. subclavian vein
29. extended and internally rotated 30 degrees
30. A. common iliac artery
   B. external iliac artery
   C. profunda femoris artery
   D. femoral artery
   E. popliteal artery
   F. anterior tibial artery
   G. peroneal artery
   H. posterior tibial artery
31. ankle
32. for force filling of the deep veins of the leg
33. 3
34. to serve as a subtraction mask

35. arterial, capillary, and venous
36. a. capillary
    b. arterial
    c. venous
37. infraorbitomeatal
38. caudally
39. away from the injected side
40. cephalically

Self-Test: Anatomy and Radiography of the Circulatory System

1. c	6. b	11. a	16. d
2. d	7. a	12. a	17. b
3. c	8. b	13. c	18. a
4. a	9. a	14. c	19. b
5. d	10. b	15. c	20. d

Chapter 27: Sectional Anatomy for Radiographers

Chapter 27 Review

1. A. frontal bone
   B. superior sagittal sinus
   C. parietal bone
   D. white matter
   E. falx cerebri (longitudinal fissure)
2. A. genu of corpus callosum
   B. internal capsule
   C. basal nuclei
   D. third ventricle
   E. occipital lobe
   F. longitudinal fissure
   G. anterior horn of lateral ventricle
   H. caudate nucleus
   I. thalamus
   J. posterior horn of lateral ventricle
3. A. longitudinal fissure
   B. middle cerebral artery
   C. basilar artery
   D. pons
   E. fourth ventricle
   F. cerebellum
   G. frontal lobe
   H. frontal sinus
   I. anterior cerebral artery
   J. posterior cerebral artery
   K. mastoid air cells
4. A. sphenoidal sinus
   B. internal carotid artery
   C. pars petrosa
   D. auricle of ear
   E. ethmoidal air cells
   F. ocular bulb
   G. optic nerve

H. temporal lobe
I. basilar artery
J. pons
K. cerebellum
5. A. mandibular symphysis
   B. hyoid
   C. submandibular gland
   D. common carotid artery
   E. sternocleidomastoid muscle
   F. internal jugular vein
   G. epiglottic cartilage
   H. laryngopharynx
6. A. common carotid artery
   B. thyroid gland
   C. thyroid cartilage
   D. larynx
   E. pharynx
   F. internal jugular vein
   G. trapezius muscle
   H. body of T6
   I. vertebral artery
7. A. lateral ventricle
   B. third ventricle
   C. optic chiasm
   D. hypophysis cerebri (pituitary gland)
   E. sphenoidal sinus
   F. clivus
   G. nasopharynx
   H. maxilla
   I. tongue
   J. corpus callosum
   K. great cerebral vein (of Galen)
   L. corpora quadrigemina
   M. cerebral aqueduct
   N. straight sinus
   O. cerebellum
   P. fourth ventricle
   Q. pons
   R. basilar artery
   S. cervical spinal cord
   T. second cervical vertebra
8. A. superior sagittal sinus
   B. longitudinal fissure
   C. corpus callosum
   D. lateral ventricle
   E. septum pellucidum
   F. lateral fissure
   G. sphenoidal sinus
   H. mandibular ramus
   I. masseter muscle
   J. submandibular gland
   K. caudate nucleus
   L. basal nuclei
   M. third ventricle
   N. optic chiasm
   O. hypophysis cerebri

P. internal carotid artery
Q. nasopharynx
R. medial pterygoid muscle
S. oropharynx
9. A. superior sagittal sinus
   B. lateral ventricle
   C. third ventricle
   D. external acoustic canal
   E. parotid gland
   F. dens
   G. vertebral artery
   H. internal carotid artery
   I. thalamus
   J. cranial nerves (in internal acoustic canal)
   K. sternocleidomastoid muscle
10. A. lateral ventricle
    B. pineal body
    C. superior and inferior colliculi
    D. pinna
    E. middle cerebellar peduncle
    F. medulla oblongata
    G. cervical spinal cord
    H. corpus callosum (splenium)
    I. cerebral aqueduct
    J. cerebellum
    K. mastoid region
11. A. manubrium
    B. brachiocephalic artery
    C. right brachiocephalic vein
    D. trachea
    E. esophagus
    F. scapula
    G. left common carotid artery
    H. left brachiocephalic vein
    I. left subclavian artery
    J. left lung
12. A. sternum
    B. ascending aorta
    C. superior vena cava
    D. right pulmonary artery
    E. right primary bronchus
    F. azygos vein
    G. body of T5
    H. pulmonary trunk
    I. left pulmonary artery
    J. descending aorta
    K. scapula
13. **A. serratus anterior muscle**
    B. liver
    C. right atrium
    D. right ventricle
    E. sternum
    F. left ventricle
    G. esophagus
    H. latissimus dorsi muscle
    I. descending aorta

J. azygos vein
K. inferior vena cava
14. A. pharynx
    B. tongue
    C. epiglottis
    D. trachea
    E. left brachiocephalic vein
    F. manubrium
    G. C2 vertebra
    H. spinal cord
    I. intervertebral disk
    J. brachiocephalic artery
    K. aortic arch
    L. right pulmonary artery
15. A. spinal cord
    B. sternocleidomastoid muscle
    C. right lung
    D. tracheal bifurcation
    E. heart
    F. left subclavian artery
    G. clavicle
    H. acromion
    I. humeral head
    J. aortic arch
    K. pulmonary trunk
16. A. liver
    B. lower lobe of right lung
    C. stomach
    D. diaphragm
    E. spleen
    F. esophagus
    G. aorta
17. A. caudate lobe
    B. right lobe of liver
    C. portal vein
    D. quadrate lobe
    E. ligamentum teres
    F. left lobe of liver
    G. stomach
    H. aorta
    I. spleen
    J. crus of diaphragm
    K. inferior vena cava
18. A. superior mesenteric artery
    B. right lobe of liver
    C. inferior vena cava
    D. right kidney
    E. crus of diaphragm
    F. stomach
    G. rectus abdominis muscle
    H. body of pancreas
    I. left colic (splenic) flexure
    J. aorta
19. A. inferior vena cava
    B. right lobe of liver
    C. aorta

D. left kidney

E. stomach (with contrast)

F. tail of pancreas

G. spleen

20. A. psoas major muscle

B. iliacus (iliac) muscle

C. ureter

D. rectus abdominis muscle

E. anterior superior iliac spine (ASIS)

F. ilium

G. sacroiliac (SI) joint

21. A. femoral vessels

B. symphysis pubis

C. bladder

D. acetabulum

E. head of femur

F. rectum

G. gluteus

22. A. obturator externus muscle

B. obturator internus muscle

C. greater trochanter

D. prostate

E. rectum

F. spermatic cord

G. corpora cavernosa (of penis)

H. pubic bone

I. femoral vessels

J. femoral head

K. gluteus maximus muscle

L. ischium

23. A. aorta

B. rectus abdominis muscle

C. bladder

D. pubic bone

E. corpora cavernosa

F. cauda equina

G. L4 vertebra

H. sacrum

I. rectum

J. coccyx

K. prostatic urethra (within prostate)

L. corpus spongiosum

M. testicles (testes)

24. A. sigmoid colon

B. bladder

C. ductus deferens

D. prostate

E. gracilis muscle

F. psoas muscle

G. iliacus (iliac) muscle

H. ilium

I. gluteus medius muscle

J. gluteus minimus muscle

K. acetabulum

L. pubic ramus

M. corpus spongiosum

N. scrotum

Appendix: Supplemental Exercises for Skull Positioning

Skull Positioning Review

Exercise 1

1. p
2. o
3. n
4. c
5. f
6. m
7. j
8. f
9. m
10. i
11. b
12. e
13. a
14. a
15. f

Exercise 2

1. g
2. b
3. n
4. e
5. d
6. m
7. p
8. o
9. a
10. f
11. c
12. j
13. h
14. k
15. l

Exercise 3

1. A
2. J
3. K
4. H
5. N
6. F
7. I
8. G
9. D
10. H
11. R
12. E
13. M
14. M
15. S
16. H
17. H

18. P
19. Q
20. K
21. O
22. B
23. C
24. O
25. S

Self-Test: Osteology, Arthrology, and Positioning of the Skull

1. c	33. d	65. b	97. a
2. d	34. b	66. c	98. d
3. a	35. b	67. c	99. c
4. b	36. b	68. b	100. c
5. c	37. a	69. a	101. a
6. d	38. a	70. a	102. b
7. d	39. b	71. d	103. a
8. d	40. a	72. a	104. a
9. a	41. b	73. d	105. b
10. b	42. d	74. d	106. c
11. c	43. b	75. a	107. d
12. d	44. c	76. b	108. c
13. a	45. b	77. d	109. b
14. c	46. c	78. b	110. c
15. a	47. b	79. d	111. d
16. b	48. a	80. a	112. a
17. a	49. c	81. d	113. a
18. c	50. c	82. c	114. a
19. b	51. a	83. a	115. a
20. c	52. c	84. b	116. c
21. d	53. d	85. a	117. c
22. b	54. d	86. c	118. a
23. a	55. c	87. a	119. d
24. b	56. c	88. b	120. b
25. a	57. d	89. a	121. c
26. c	58. a	90. b	122. c
27. d	59. b	91. c	123. b
28. d	60. c	92. c	124. b
29. a	61. d	93. a	125. a
30. c	62. d	94. b	
31. d	63. b	95. c	
32. d	64. c	96. a	